Frye's

3300

Nursing
Bullets

NCLEX-PN®

FOURTH EDITION

Charles M. Frye, RN, MEd, JD

President
West Haven University
Salt Lake City, Utah

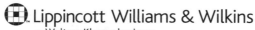

Lippincott Williams & Wilkins
a Wolters Kluwer business
Philadelphia · Baltimore · New York · London
Buenos Aires · Hong Kong · Sydney · Tokyo

STAFF

Executive Publisher
Judith A. Schilling McCann, RN, MSN

Editorial Directors
H. Nancy Holmes, William J. Kelly

Clinical Director
Joan M. Robinson, RN, MSN

Art Director
Elaine Kasmer

Editorial Project Manager
Sean Webb

Editors
Toby H. Brener, Catherine E. Harold,
Patricia Nale

Copy Editors
Kimberly Bilotta (supervisor),
Shana Harrington, Dona Hightower
Perkins, Pamela Wingrod

Digital Composition Services
Diane Paluba (manager),
Joyce Rossi Biletz, Donald G. Knauss

Manufacturing
Beth J. Welsh

Editorial Assistants
Megan L. Aldinger, Karen J. Kirk,
Linda K. Ruhf

Indexer
Barbara Hodgson

The clinical procedures described and recommended in this publication are based on research and consultation with nursing, medical, and legal authorities. To the best of our knowledge, these procedures reflect currently accepted practice; nevertheless, they can't be considered absolute and universal recommendations. For individual application, all recommendations must be considered in light of the patient's clinical condition and, before administration of new or infrequently used drugs, in light of the latest package-insert information. The authors and the publisher disclaim responsibility for any adverse effects resulting directly or indirectly from the suggested procedures, from any undetected errors, or from the reader's misunderstanding of the text.

NCLEX-PN® is a registered trademark of the National Council of State Boards of Nursing, Inc.

FBPN011106—090313

Library of Congress Cataloging-in-Publication Data

Frye, Charles M.
Frye's 3300 nursing bullets NCLEX-PN / Charles M. Frye. — 4th ed.
        p. ; cm.
    Includes index.
    Rev. ed. of: Frye's 3000 nursing bullets NCLEX-PN. 3rd ed. c2004.
    1. Practical nursing — Examinations, questions, etc. 2. Practical nursing — Outlines, syllabi, etc. 3. National Council Licensure Examination for Practical/Vocational Nurses — Study guides I. Frye, Charles M. Frye's 3000 nursing bullets NCLEX-PN. II. Title. III. Title: 3300 nursing bullets NCLEX-PN. IV. Title: NCLEX-PN. V. Title: Frye's thirty-three hundred nursing bullets NCLEX-PN.
    [DNLM: 1. Nursing, Practical — Examination Questions. WY 18.2F948f 2007]
    RT62.F793 2007
    ISBN13: 978-1-58255-463-1
    ISBN10: 1-58255-463-3 (alk. paper)   2006025705

Contents

Dedicated to my two wonderful sons,
Randall and Shawn.
You two not only add meaning to my life,
you are my life.

Contributors and consultants

Elizabeth (Libby) A. Archer,
RN, EdDc
Assistant Professor
Baptist College of Health
Sciences
Memphis

Marsha L. Conroy RN, MSN, APN
Nursing Educator
Cuyahoga Community College
Cleveland

Charlene K. Eshleman, RN, BSN,
MSN
Clinical Nurse Specialist
Lancaster (Pa.) Regional Medical
Center

Mercy Flynn, RN
Coordinator, Instructor in
Nursing
Christus Spohn Hospital, Coastal
Bend College
Beeville, Tex.

Connie S. Heflin, RN, MSN
Professor of Nursing
Paducah (Ky.) Community
Hospital

Shelton M. Hisley, RNC, PhD,
WHNP
Assistant Professor of Nursing
The University of North Carolina
at Wilmington

Gwendolyn L. Jordan, RN, MSN
Carolinas College of Health
Sciences
Charlotte, N.C.

Theresa Pulvano, RN, BSN
LPN Nursing Educator
Ocean County Vocational
Technical School
Toms River, N.J.

Student Reviewers

Christine Hoener, LPN
RN Nursing Student
Cochise College
Sierra Vista, Ariz.

Manuel Marquez, AS
Nursing Student
Pace University
Pleasantville, N.Y.

Preface

In the more than 300 nursing review seminars that I have conducted, one thing is certain—when it comes to preparing for examinations, nursing candidates don't want to waste time learning things they don't need to know.

Unfortunately, no one knows with any certainty what will be on the next NCLEX-PN® examination. Generally, candidates try to learn everything. They over-study certain areas, under-study others, and neglect the rest.

This is where *Frye's 3300 Nursing Bullets NCLEX-PN®*, Fourth Edition, can make a difference. It's designed as a quick reference to numerous nursing procedures and disease processes, ideas on taking the NCLEX-PN, and tidbits of information that routinely surface on the examination.

This book is also ideal for nursing students; they can refer to it as they progress through their programs. It offers a condensed view of the nursing program packed into an easy-to-carry book.

How to use this book

Frye's 3300 Nursing Bullets NCLEX-PN®, Fourth Edition, is designed to help you review for the NCLEX-PN® effectively and efficiently. This book gives you nursing information for every clinical situation and setting—the very facts that question writers must draw on in devising the test.

Follow these suggestions to get the most from this unique book:

▶ Read the introduction to prepare for computerized adaptive testing, learn about the NCLEX-PN test plan, and develop effective test-taking strategies.

▶ Study the key facts as they're presented in random order. You'll realize two benefits from this approach: You'll master essential data in psychiatric, pediatric, maternal, and medical-surgical nursing as well as the important concepts in nursing fundamentals, and you'll prepare yourself for the computerized NCLEX-PN, which also presents questions in a random style. (After each bulleted fact in this book, the applicable clinical topic area appears in parentheses: FND for fundamentals, MAT for maternal-neonatal nursing, M-S for medical-surgical nursing, PED for pediatric nursing, and PSY for psychiatric nursing.)

▶ Review groups of nursing bullets throughout the day. Because this book is compact and easy to carry, you can take it with you wherever you go and review a few bullets whenever you have a spare minute—while waiting for class to begin, during a break between labs, or while riding the bus or train.

▶ Use the book to create questions to quiz your study partner or members of your study group.

No matter how you choose to use this versatile book, you'll find that each nursing bullet is brief, easy to read, and free from distracting clinical situations and excess wording. You'll find that you'll easily remember and identify the facts, no matter what form they take on the test. Because each bullet has been reviewed by a clinical expert, you can be sure that all the information is up-to-date and clinically accurate.

You've spent years studying to become a nurse and months preparing for the NCLEX-PN. Now, with *Frye's 3300 Nursing Bullets NCLEX-PN®*, Fourth Edition, you can take the last step to licensure with confidence. Please note, though, that this book is intended to serve as a study aid. Because of the abbreviated information about diseases, processes, and nursing interventions, it shouldn't be used as a guide to clinical practice.

Introduction

In the United States, if you want to work as a licensed practical nurse, you need a license from the nursing licensure authority in the state where you plan to practice. To get a license, you need to pass the National Council Licensure Examination for Practical Nurses (NCLEX-PN®). This book will help you do just that. Its 3,300 bullets of nursing facts will expand and reinforce your nursing knowledge base. This introduction will prepare you for the examination by describing computerized adaptive testing, explaining the NCLEX-PN test plan, and providing effective test-taking strategies.

Scheduling your test

To schedule your NCLEX-PN, apply to your state board of nursing for testing. When your application is approved, the Educational Testing Service Data Center will send you an Authorization to Test and will advise you to make an examination appointment at one of the Pearson VUE Centers located throughout the country.

When scheduling your NCLEX-PN, remember that the test takes up to 5 hours and is offered 15 hours daily, Monday through Saturday, and sometimes on Sunday. The Pearson VUE Center will schedule you for testing within 30 days of your call (or within 45 days for retesting). If you need to reschedule your examination appointment, call the Pearson VUE Center at least 24 hours beforehand.

Understanding computerized adaptive testing

Since April of 1994, the NCLEX-PN has been a computerized test. It requires you to answer a sufficient number of questions of various levels of difficulty to demonstrate minimum competence as an entry-level nurse. It's adaptive because it selects harder or easier questions based on your response to previous questions. For example, if you answer a medium-level question correctly, the computer will pose a more difficult question next. If you answer incorrectly, it will choose an easier one.

The test bank includes thousands of questions categorized by level of difficulty and the NCLEX-PN test plan. From this bank, the computer continues to pull questions until you demonstrate competence in all parts of the test plan. Therefore, each test is different and may require 85 to 205 questions to complete.

Before the test, a proctor will help you get started at a computer terminal. The test will begin with a brief tutorial that reviews the different types of questions that appear on the test and 15 pretest questions. During the test you may use the mouse or the number keyboard to select your answer. To avoid unintentional answers, the computer will ask you to confirm your answer selection.

During the test, the computer will display one question at a time. Because the computer doesn't let you skip questions or return to previous items, you must answer every question until the test ends. The testing period includes two optional 10-minute breaks, the first one after 2 hours and the second one after 3½ hours.

Understanding the NCLEX-PN test plan
The NCLEX-PN test plan classifies questions by the steps of the nursing process and the categories of client needs. Each test question reflects one nursing process step and one client needs category.

Nursing process steps
The nursing process is a four-step method of performing nursing care. On the NCLEX-PN, each nursing process step carries equal weight.

▶ *Data collection* refers to forming a database by gathering subjective and objective information about a client.

▶ *Planning* refers to establishing goals to meet the client's needs and developing strategies for achieving those goals.

▶ *Implementation* refers to performing actions that accomplish the client's established goals.

▶ *Evaluation* refers to measuring the extent of goal achievement.

Client needs
The health needs of clients are organized by four major categories that were identified during a 1997 job analysis study of newly licensed practical nurses. The four categories are safe, effective care environment; health promotion and maintenance; psychosocial integrity; and physiological integrity.

Safe, effective care environment
- Coordinated care (11% to 17% of the test)
  - Providing integrated, cost-effective care to clients by coordinating, supervising, or collaborating with members of the multidisciplinary health care team
- Safety and infection control (8% to 14% of the test)
  - Protecting clients and health care personnel from environmental hazards

Health promotion and maintenance (7% to 13% of the test)

Psychosocial integrity (8% to 14% of the test)

Physiological integrity
- Basic care and comfort (11% to 17% of the test)

- Providing comfort and assistance in the performance of activities of daily living
- Pharmacological therapies (9% to 15% of the test)
  - Managing and providing care related to the administration of medications
- Reduction of risk potential (10% to 16% of the test)
  - Reducing the likelihood that clients will develop complications or health problems related to existing conditions, treatments, or procedures
- Physiological adaptation (12% to 18% of the test)
  - Managing and providing care to clients who have acute, chronic, or life-threatening physical health conditions

Studying for the examination

To study for the NCLEX-PN as effectively as possible and enhance your ability to retain pertinent information, follow these study tips:

▶ Familiarize yourself with all examination topics.

▶ Answer as many practice questions as possible. (You may want to use this book's bullets to develop questions with a study partner.)

▶ Understand the parts of a test question. On the NCLEX-PN, each multiple-choice question has a stem (the question itself) and four options: a key (correct answer) and three distracters (incorrect answers). A brief case study may precede any question. New alternate-format questions may also include multiple-choice items in which there may be more than one correct response, fill in the blank, chart-exhibit questions, drag and drop items, or items asking a candidate to identify an area on a picture or graphic. Any item formats may include tables, charts, or graphic images.

▶ Use additional study guides as resources, such as the *Springhouse Review for NCLEX-PN*, if desired.

▶ Organize a study group with other nursing students or take an NCLEX review course.

▶ Ask a colleague or nursing instructor to clarify unfamiliar or complex material.

Planning for the examination

Remember that the NCLEX-PN poses certain physical demands. To cope with these demands, ensure your best test performance, and help you plan for the examination, use these pointers:

▶ Schedule your test appointment at a testing center near your home, if possible. Before the test, assess the parking facilities and determine travel time.

▶ Make reservations well in advance at a hotel near the testing center if you must travel a long distance.

▶ Schedule your test appointment to take advantage of your peak-performance time.

▶ Avoid late-night, last-minute cramming. Obtain sufficient sleep the night before the test.

▶ Eat a well-balanced meal before the test.

▶ Wear layers of clothes that can be removed, as needed, to keep you comfortable.

▶ Take your Authorization to Test and two forms of identification with signatures (including one photographic identification) to the testing center. You can't take the examination without them.

▶ Use simple relaxation techniques, such as progressive relaxation, during the test to reduce anxiety.

Developing test-taking skills

Knowing the facts isn't all you need to pass the NCLEX-PN. You also need to know how to take the test. To sharpen your test-taking skills, review these guidelines:

▶ Check case studies closely for information needed to answer the question correctly.

▶ Look for clue words, such as *best, first, most,* and *not* in the question's stem. These words, which may be highlighted, aid in selecting the correct answer.

▶ Imagine the correct response when reading the stem. If it appears as one of the four options, it's probably the correct one.

▶ Read every question—and all four of its options—carefully before making your final selection.

▶ Reread the stem and options when two options seem equally correct; look again for clues or differences that can help you select the correct answer. When in doubt, make an educated guess. Remember: You can't skip questions.

▶ Don't panic if a question covers an unfamiliar topic. Draw on your knowledge of similar problems and nursing principles to help eliminate options and increase the chance of choosing the correct answer.

▶ Take your time and pace yourself. Don't spend excessive time on any one question.

▶ Don't be distracted by other candidates or the apparent length of their tests. Keep in mind that each test is individualized.

▶ Use break periods to rest your mind and body—for example, eat a small snack, stretch, or do relaxation exercises.

Frye's
3300
Nursing
Bullets

NCLEX-PN®

FOURTH EDITION

▶ When inserting a suppository, unless contraindicated, place a client on his left side with the right knee flexed. **(FND)**

▶ When developing any therapeutic program, the client's preferences are always a priority and should be considered. **(FND)**

▶ There are no restrictions on how a client with a colostomy should bathe. **(FND)**

▶ When bottle-feeding a neonate with a cleft palate, hold the infant's head in an upright position. **(PED)**

▶ Because circulating maternal antibodies decrease an immune response, the measles, mumps, and rubella (MMR) vaccine shouldn't be given until the infant is 1 year old. **(PED)**

▶ If a client has sustained trauma to the hand or arm, remove jewelry items, such as rings, watches, and bracelets, to prevent constriction if edema develops. **(M-S)**

▶ Recognizing the differences between one's own culture and the culture of another is called *cultural awareness*. **(FND)**

▶ Complications associated with systemic lupus erythematosus are renal failure, neurologic dysfunction, and death. **(M-S)**

▶ *Stereotyping* is the assumption that people of a specific sect, group, community, or race will act or respond in a specific manner or have the same traits. For example, telling a client "most people don't experience that level of pain during the procedure" is stereotyping. **(FND)**

▶ When the family wants to involve a faith healer in the client's care, the first thing the nurse should do is ask the family what the faith healer plans to do. The nurse can then share the family's wishes with the physician. **(FND)**

▶ Call clients by their last name (using Mr., Mrs., Ms., Dr.) until given permission to do otherwise. **(FND)**

▶ If a client has increased pain when the testicle is palpated, suspect testicular torsion; if he's relieved when the scrotum is lifted, suspect epididymitis. **(M-S)**

▶ A *standing order* is a written policy, regulation, order, or rule that provides specific guidance on how to handle a particular treatment issue, problem, or concern. **(FND)**

▶ Four steps in developing a care plan are to set priorities, establish client goals and desired outcomes, identify nursing interventions, and write corresponding nursing orders. **(FND)**

▶ A nurse blocks effective communication with a client if she gives common advice, challenges the client, makes a value judgment, changes the topic of discussion, or gives approval or disapproval of the client's actions. **(FND)**

▶ When caring for a client with a cognitive disorder, such as Alzheimer's disease or dementia, the nurse should frequently orient the client to time, place, and person; provide continuity of care and consistent routines; provide activities to stimulate the client; provide encouragement and assist in a step-by-step fashion if necessary; and place familiar objects such as a favorite chair or pictures of loved ones in the client's room. **(M-S)**

▶ The desire to acquire the sexual characteristics of the opposite sex is called *transsexualism.* **(PSY)**

▶ The leading cause of Laënnec's cirrhosis in the United States is alcohol abuse. **(M-S)**

▶ The typical sign of an inguinal hernia is protrusion of a mass in the groin. **(M-S)**

▶ Boneless, skinless baked chicken is low in fat and triglycerides. **(FND)**

▶ An incomplete protein lacks one or more of the essential amino acids and is usually derived from plants. **(FND)**

▶ Fiber is a complex carbohydrate that can't be digested and adds bulk to the diet. **(FND)**

▶ *Glycogenesis* is the process of forming glycogen from glucose. **(FND)**

▶ Nitrogen balance occurs when nitrogen intake equals output. **(FND)**

▶ Transferrin transports iron from the intestine into the blood. **(FND)**

▶ A common adverse effect of antibiotic use is diarrhea. **(FND)**

▶ During a nasogastric (NG) tube feeding, the head of the bed should be elevated for about 30 minutes to aid in the absorption process. **(FND)**

▶ After an NG tube feeding, flush the NG tube with water. Add the amount of water to the intake and output record. **(FND)**

▶ The appropriate diagnosis for a client who has been incontinent would be *Risk for impaired skin integrity related to frequent contact with feces and urine* and the appropriate diagnosis for a client on prolonged bed rest would be *Risk for impaired skin integrity related to prolonged bed rest.* **(FND)**

▶ As oxygen level decreases, the client will advance to a stupor state. **(M-S)**

▶ Behavior modification is one method used to treat an obese client. **(M-S)**

▶ Typical signs of dehydration in an infant are a depressed or sunken fontanel, sunken eyeballs, decreased tearing, and poor skin turgor. **(PED)**

▶ In a kosher diet, meat and dairy products—for example, a cheeseburger—can't be eaten together. **(FND)**

▶ To achieve postural drainage in an infant, place a pillow on the nurse's lap then lay the infant across it. **(PED)**

▶ Glycerin suppositories are given 30 minutes before expected defecation time. **(FND)**

▶ To avoid postural hypotension in a client taking a loop diuretic, have the client sit on the edge of the bed and dangle his feet before standing. **(FND)**

▶ Pale-colored or clear urine or low concentration may indicate overhydration. **(FND)**

▶ In a client with pneumothorax, breath sounds are diminished or absent on the affected side during auscultation. **(M-S)**

 ▶ A child with cystic fibrosis should consume more calories, protein, vitamins, and minerals than a child without the disease. **(PED)**

▶ Sodium polystyrene sulfonate is a potassium-removing resin used as medication for clients with hyperkalemia. **(M-S)**

▶ A potassium elixir is mixed or dissolved in water, then drunk slowly. **(FND)**

▶ The most dangerous electrolyte abnormality in chronic renal failure is hyperkalemia. **(M-S)**

▶ Most food absorption takes place in the small intestine. **(FND)**

▶ When giving a nasogastric tube feeding, the nursing priority is to check placement. **(FND)**

▶ In clients with diabetes insipidus, the nurse should monitor urine output and check urine specific gravity. **(M-S)**

▶ Before a barium enema test is given, the client's large bowel is thoroughly cleaned to promote visualization. **(M-S)**

▶ Expect bowel sounds to return within 12 to 24 hours after abdominal surgery. **(M-S)**

▶ The most effective method of increasing oral fluid intake is to frequently offer small amounts of favorite fluids. **(FND)**

▶ Older clients don't need as many calories as younger clients because they aren't as active. **(FND)**

▶ The salicylate in aspirin and ibuprofen can irritate gastric mucosa, especially in clients with peptic ulcer disease. **(M-S)**

▶ Processed fruits and vegetables have more sodium than fresh fruits and vegetables. **(FND)**

▶ Bile is produced in the liver and stored in the gallbladder. The liver produces 600 to 1,200 ml of bile every day. **(FND)**

▶ Bile is needed to metabolize fat. When bile is blocked or not produced in sufficient quantity, a typical clinical manifestation is fatty, bulky stools. **(FND)**

▶ Don't give a client with abdominal pain any pain medication until a diagnosis is made because it may mask more serious complications.   **(M-S)**

▶ To prevent aspiration in a client receiving continuous nasogastric tube feedings, place the client in a reverse Trendelenburg (head upward) position.   **(FND)**

▶ The expected intervention for an infant with pyloric stenosis is surgery.   **(PED)**

▶ A client of the Islamic faith won't consume pork.   **(FND)**

▶ Rickets is caused by a vitamin D deficiency.   **(M-S)**

▶ Infants subsisting on cow's milk only don't receive a sufficient amount of iron (ferrous sulfate), and will eventually show signs of iron deficiency anemia.   **(PED)**

▶ Painless enlargement of the testicle is the typical first sign of testicular cancer.   **(M-S)**

▶ Gentamicin sulfate (Garamycin) is ototoxic and can cause hearing loss.   **(FND)**

▶ To prevent exposure to rubella, a pregnant nurse shouldn't work in a pediatric setting.   **(MAT)**

▶ In vitro exposure to rubella can harm the fetus, resulting in deafness, heart murmurs, or cataracts.   **(MAT)**

▶ Hepatitis A vaccine (HAV) administered before exposure to the virus effectively prevents the development of the disease.   **(M-S)**

▶ Use lotion and lanolin cream on a donor site to keep the site soft and minimize scarring.   **(M-S)**

▶ Only the epidermis is affected in a partial-thickness (first-degree) burn.   **(M-S)**

▶ The transdermal method has the slowest absorption rate of all methods of administering medication.   **(FND)**

▶ The bacterium that causes acne is *Propionibacterium acnes*.   **(M-S)**

▶ Mongolian spots are common in dark-skinned clients and usually disappear with age.   **(M-S)**

▶ Erythema in a dark-skinned client appears dusky red or violet; in a light-skinned client, erythema appears diffusely red.   **(FND)**

▶ Expect substantial bleeding in the hours after abdominal surgery. In the days after surgery, bleeding should advance from sanguineous to serosanguineous to serous.   **(M-S)**

► Steroidal bronchodilators increase the client's risk of infection because of a compromised immune system. Have clients rinse their mouth to reduce the risk of acquiring an oral fungal infection. **(FND)**

► Clients who have had cataract extraction should move their head slowly to avoid increasing intraocular pressure. **(M-S)**

► A prosthetic artificial eye should be placed in water and stored in the plastic container in which it was issued. The fluid doesn't need to be sterile. **(FND)**

► Clients receiving corticosteroids for conditions such as nephritic syndrome should be monitored for signs of infection. Any sign should be reported immediately to the attending physician. **(FND)**

► Before undergoing abdominal paracentesis, the client should void to minimize the risk of rupturing the bladder. **(M-S)**

► Contributing to the relatively low failure rate of oral contraceptives is failure to take the medication as prescribed. **(MAT)**

► Breast-feeding mothers should increase calcium and protein in their diet. **(MAT)**

► Nursing interventions that cause pain should be clustered to minimize the frequency of painful experiences. **(FND)**

► Activities should be paced with clients prone to activity intolerance. **(FND)**

► The nurse shouldn't record respirations, pulse, or blood pressure when a client is crying; the measurements will likely be falsely elevated. **(FND)**

► When a client is receiving oxygen via a mask, don't obtain the client's temperature orally. **(FND)**

► Don't take an oral temperature in a confused or crying client. **(FND)**

► Glucocorticoids promote sodium retention, so a client receiving such treatment should be on a low-sodium diet. **(FND)**

► Tenderness is a common finding after bone marrow biopsy; treat it with a mild analgesic. **(FND)**

► Rocky Mountain spotted fever is transmitted by the bite of a tick; symptoms include prolonged fever and headaches. **(M-S)**

► *Haemophilus influenzae* type b vaccine is administered to children and infants to prevent bacterial pneumonia, bacterial meningitis, sepsis, and epiglottitis. **(PED)**

► The initial treatment for a client with hemarthrosis (bleeding within a joint) is immobilization with the joint slightly flexed. **(M-S)**

▶ Before pouring a sterile solution contained within a clean container into a sterile receptacle, the nurse should pour a small amount out to clean the lip. **(FND)**

▶ A child with an undiagnosed infection should be placed in isolation. **(PED)**

▶ A pregnant woman with sickle cell anemia needs supplemental iron to maintain iron stores and enhance the oxygen-carrying capacity of the blood by increasing the hemoglobin. **(MAT)**

▶ The initial and continuing assessment of a client who has suffered a dislocation includes assessing pulsations below the level of the dislocation. **(M-S)**

▶ Because a nurse should assess before carrying out any activity, when selecting an answer to a question on the examination, look for the choices that "assess" the client's condition. Assessment doesn't mean inaction. Assessment includes taking vital signs, asking questions, inspecting for outward signs and symptoms, and using the senses to evaluate the client. **(FND)**

▶ Unless ordered, a nurse doesn't allow family members or friends to provide treatment, such as administering medication, changing a wound dressing, or suctioning a client. **(FND)**

▶ The best way to determine the client's customs, traditions, and religious beliefs is to ask the client. **(FND)**

▶ The classic signs and symptoms of meningitis are nuchal rigidity, severe headache, and high temperature. **(M-S)**

▶ Protect the personal belongings of deceased clients. If a person takes any item belonging to the client, note what was taken in the chart. **(FND)**

▶ Only the client can rate his own pain. **(FND)**

▶ If the physician writes an order for pain medication as needed, the nurse can't refuse the client's request for the medication. **(FND)**

▶ Documentation of delivered care is the best defense against a malpractice claim. **(FND)**

▶ The diagonal conjugate is about 1½" (3.8 cm) larger than the obstetrical conjugate. **(MAT)**

▶ A pregnant client shouldn't use sodium bicarbonate for heartburn because sodium bicarbonate may alter the electrolyte balance. **(MAT)**

▶ A low enema is used to clean the sigmoid colon and the rectum. **(FND)**

▶ The normal urine output for an adult client is 1,500 ml per day. **(FND)**

▶ A symptom of an enlarged prostate is urinary urgency and frequency. **(M-S)**

▶ A client with a urinary catheter should take a shower rather than a tub bath to decrease the risk of bacteria ascending to the bladder via the catheter tubing. **(FND)**

▶ To prevent damage to the urethra when inserting a catheter in a male client, straighten the penis so that it's perpendicular to the body. **(FND)**

▶ Clients with neurogenic bladder dysfunction are candidates for clean intermittent self-catheterization (CISC). **(M-S)**

▶ The most common urinary diversion is an ileal conduit or ileal loop. **(M-S)**

▶ The medulla and the pons control respiration. **(FND)**

▶ A high percentage (65%) of carbon dioxide is transported from the cells to the lungs via red blood cells in the form of bicarbonate. About one-half of that amount (30%) combines with hemoglobin. **(FND)**

▶ The two bed positions that provide the greatest expansion of the lungs are the semi-Fowler and high Fowler positions. **(FND)**

▶ A nebulizer delivers oxygen and medication. **(FND)**

▶ If a nonrebreather mask's reservoir is collapsed, immediately remove the mask and assess respiration; provide ventilatory support as required. (A client isn't getting any air or oxygen if the reservoir collapses.) **(FND)**

▶ The four routes of fluid output are urine, feces, insensible losses (through lungs and skin), and sweat. **(FND)**

▶ Buffers prevent excessive changes in the pH of the blood by releasing and removing hydrogen ions. **(FND)**

▶ The major buffers in the extracellular fluid are bicarbonate and carbonic acid. **(FND)**

▶ The four main blood groups are types A, B, AB, and O. **(FND)**

▶ Stop a client from performing a therapeutic activity if the client complains of dizziness, weakness, or shortness of breath or if the client has a change in heart rate or respiratory rate, or a weakening of the pulse. **(FND)**

▶ Alternatives to meat for a vegetarian client are soybean curds, meat analogs, and textured soy protein. **(FND)**

▶ A client taking Procardia (nifedipine) shouldn't consume grapefruit because of the risk of toxicity. **(FND)**

▶ A high-fat diet is associated with colon cancer. **(FND)**

▶ A high-protein, high-calorie diet is recommended for a client with cystic fibrosis. **(PED)**

▶ Eggs are an appropriate food for a low-residue diet. **(FND)**

▶ A client with lactose intolerance should avoid milk and cheese.   (FND)

▶ Vitamins, fat, and protein are delivered via total parenteral nutrition (TPN).
     (FND)

▶ To reduce the risk of constipation, the client should consume a high-fiber diet.
     (FND)

▶ Vegetable sources of iron include spinach, kidney beans, and soybeans.
     (FND)

▶ A vegetarian diet is high in fiber.   (FND)

▶ Alcohol consumption in the absence of food intake can cause hypoglycemia.
     (FND)

▶ The mucus in the large intestine protects the intestinal wall from bacteria and fecal acid.   (FND)

▶ An elderly client is predisposed to constipation because of a loss of tonus of the smooth muscles in the colon.   (FND)

▶ Paralytic ileus is the temporary cessation of intestinal movement after surgery. The client is maintained nothing-by-mouth until bowel sounds return.
     (M-S)

▶ Protracted diarrhea can cause fluid and electrolyte imbalance.   (M-S)

▶ Water intoxication can occur in clients receiving a hypotonic enema. (FND)

▶ When preparing a female client for catheterization, clean from front to back without separating the labia.   (FND)

▶ The appropriate diet for a client with Crohn's disease is a low-fat, lactose-free diet.   (M-S)

▶ A natural intestinal deodorizer is cranberry juice.   (FND)

▶ Vitamin B$_{12}$ is lacking in a vegetarian diet because it's mostly found in animal products.   (FND)

▶ Foods rich in magnesium sulfate are nuts, grains, and green leafy vegetables.
     (FND)

▶ Protein (albumin) in the urine is a sign of glomerular injury.   (M-S)

▶ Once inserted, the tubing of a retention catheter is taped to the client's leg to stabilize it and thereby avoid injury to the external urethral sphincter.
     (FND)

▶ A chest tube drainage system should be situated below the level of the chest.
     (M-S)

▶ The proper procedure to follow when questioning an order is to contact the person who wrote or issued the order.   (FND)

▶ An infant usually triples his birth weight by the end of the first year.   **(PED)**

▶ Alcohol potentiates the effects of lithium carbonate. Clients should avoid consuming alcoholic beverages while taking this medication.   **(PSY)**

▶ Possible signs and symptoms in a client who sustained a frontal lobe injury include dysfunction with affect, emotional lability, and impaired judgment.   **(PSY)**

▶ In a child with meningitis, it's appropriate to frequently assess neurologic signs such as level of consciousness, and to measure the circumference of the head because subdural effusions and obstructive hydrocephalus can develop.   **(M-S)**

▶ Clinical signs of a dehydrated infant include lethargy, irritability, dry skin, decreased tearing, decreased urine output, and increased pulse.   **(PED)**

▶ A client on heparin or warfarin (Coumadin) should shave with an electric razor and report unusual bruising.   **(M-S)**

▶ Expected clinical findings in a neonate with cerebral palsy include reflexive hypertonicity and crisscrossing or scissoring leg movements.   **(MAT)**

▶ The fingernails of a toddler with atopic dermatitis should be trimmed.   **(PED)**

▶ Obesity in the adolescent is most commonly associated with poor body image and a lessening of self-esteem.   **(PED)**

▶ A sign of heart failure is bibasilar inspiratory crackles.   **(M-S)**

▶ Papules, vesicles, and crust are all present at the same time in the early phase of chickenpox.   **(PED)**

▶ Topical corticosteroids shouldn't be used on chickenpox lesions.   **(PED)**

▶ A client is revealing the most resistive behavior if he continues to use drugs while undergoing rehabilitation treatment.   **(PSY)**

▶ Iron deficiency anemia can occur when a toddler drinks too much milk and doesn't eat enough iron-rich foods.   **(PED)**

▶ Serving size of a food is usually 1 tablespoon for each year of age.   **(PED)**

▶ The characteristic of fifth disease (erythema infectiosum) is erythema on the face, primarily the cheeks, giving a "slapped face" appearance.   **(PED)**

▶ To assess recent memory, ask the client about (known) events that have occurred within the past 2 weeks. (It would be of little value to ask a client what he had for breakfast if the nurse didn't know what the client had for breakfast.)   **(M-S)**

▶ Adolescents may hide pain, especially in front of peers. Offer analgesics if pain is suspected or administer the medication if the client asks for it.   **(PED)**

▶ During delirium tremens, the client may experience confusion, disorientation, hypertension, extreme agitation, tremors, diaphoresis, tachycardia, and fever. **(PSY)**

▶ Signs that a child with cystic fibrosis is responding to pancreatic enzymes include absence of steatorrhea and abdominal pain, and improved appetite. **(PED)**

▶ Lidocaine shouldn't be administered unless there's continuous electrocardiographic monitoring. **(M-S)**

▶ Adverse effects of lidocaine are bradycardia, heart block, cardiovascular collapse, and cardiac arrest. **(M-S)**

▶ When teaching a client, assess his level of knowledge and learning style first. **(FND)**

▶ A stage III pressure ulcer is red (granulation of tissue) with a loss of subcutaneous tissue. **(FND)**

▶ Treatment for a stage III pressure ulcer is to clean the wound and apply a moist dressing. **(FND)**

▶ Victims of domestic violence commonly blame themselves for the abuse. **(PSY)**

▶ Inform a client taking any antibiotic of the importance of strictly complying with the physician's orders. **(FND)**

▶ Edema of the ankles that occurs during the day but disappears at night is a sign of right-sided heart failure. **(M-S)**

▶ Roseola appears as discrete rose-pink macules that first appear on the trunk and fade when pressure is applied. **(PED)**

▶ Alprazolam (Xanax) gives short-term relief of panic attacks. **(PSY)**

▶ The first action to take when a loop of umbilical cord is seen protruding from a woman in labor is to place the client in a Trendelenburg or knee-chest position. **(MAT)**

▶ Silver sulfadiazine (Silvadene) is effective against *Pseudomonas*. **(M-S)**

▶ Monitor the urine for sulfa crystals in a client receiving silver sulfadiazine (Silvadene) therapy for burns. **(M-S)**

▶ As a general rule, if the client has peripheral arterial insufficiency, place the legs in a dependent (below the heart) position. If the client has a venous return problem, elevate the legs above heart level. **(M-S)**

▶ If blood-tinged fluid is leaking from the nose and ears of a client who sustained a head injury, apply bulky, loose dressings to the ears and nose. **(M-S)**

▶ Use a needleless syringe to administer a liquid medication to an infant.
(PED)

▶ If deep vein thrombosis is suspected, place the client on bed rest until a physician can make an evaluation. (M-S)

▶ Ninety degree–ninety degree traction is used for fracture of a child's femur or tibia. (PED)

▶ The first step in alcohol treatment is to detoxify the client. (PSY)

▶ Candidiasis on the roof of a child's mouth can be distinguished from milk residue as milk can be removed with a soft cloth. (PED)

▶ Before undergoing electroconvulsive therapy, the client will need to sign an informed consent, have a spinal X-ray study, and have urine and blood samples drawn. (PSY)

▶ Undescended testis or cryptorchidism is associated with testicular cancer later in life. (M-S)

▶ To reduce the risk of trauma to the urethra, the nurse should lubricate the tip of the catheter before inserting it into a male client. (FND)

▶ Mitral insufficiency is manifested by exertional dyspnea, which is caused by fluid retention and diminished heart function. (M-S)

▶ The pathway that an impulse travels through the heart is as follows: sinoatrial (SA) node, atrioventricular (AV) node, bundle of His, and Purkinje fibers. (M-S)

▶ Gastroesophageal reflux disease is aggravated by a fatty diet, smoking, alcohol, chocolate, and meperidine (Demerol). (M-S)

▶ Stop performing passive range-of-motion exercises when the client feels pain. (FND)

▶ A nurse doesn't have to participate in euthanasia, assisted suicide, termination of life-sustaining treatment, or withdrawal or withholding of food and fluids. (FND)

▶ Passive euthanasia means removing extraordinary means of keeping a person alive (for example, discontinuing a ventilator). (FND)

▶ Advocacy involves ensuring that the client's rights are protected. (FND)

▶ One clinical sign of developmental dysplasia is limping during ambulation. (PED)

▶ Circumcision wouldn't be performed on a male child with hypospadias because the foreskin may be needed during surgical reconstruction. (MAT)

▶ Evidence of neonatal abstinence syndrome includes central nervous system hyperirritability (for example, hyperactive Moro reflex) and GI symptoms (watery stools).   **(MAT)**

▶ Atropine is contraindicated in a client with acute glaucoma and shouldn't be used to treat symptomatic bradycardia.   **(M-S)**

▶ Decreased urine outflow after a myocardial infarction is most likely attributable to decreased cardiac output.   **(M-S)**

▶ When communicating with a child 5 years old or younger, use concrete explanations.   **(PED)**

▶ To reduce stranger anxiety in children younger than age 5, have the usual caregiver assist with treatments and procedures.   **(PED)**

▶ When it's suspected that a child is being abused, the priority is to remove the child from the abusive environment to reduce the risk of further injury.   **(PED)**

▶ *Magical thinking* is a belief that simply thinking of an event will make it happen.   **(PSY)**

▶ *Osteoporosis* is a reduction in bone mass that commonly occurs in postmenopausal women.   **(M-S)**

▶ A panic disorder is characterized by shear terror, fear, and apprehension. Onset is unpredictable, although certain events, situations, or locations may precipitate an attack.   **(PSY)**

▶ A mild transient fever is expected postoperatively. A high sustained fever indicates complications: atelectasis within the first 48 hours; infection of the wound within 1 week; urinary tract infection in the first 5 days; and thrombophlebitis within the first week.   **(M-S)**

▶ Advantages to not using a dressing on a wound include better visualization of the wound; elimination of conditions that bacteria need: moistness, warmth, and darkness; and lower cost.   **(FND)**

▶ To promote nutrition in a client receiving chemotherapy, administer antiemetic therapy before administering the chemotherapeutic agent.   **(FND)**

▶ When providing care to a client with cancer, avoid invasive procedures (for example, injections) when his platelet count is less than 100,000 per cubic millimeter of blood.   **(M-S)**

▶ *Superior vena cava syndrome* is obstruction of the superior vena cava by a tumor or enlarged lymph node.   **(M-S)**

▶ Signs and symptoms of superior vena cava syndrome are facial swelling, chest pain, cough, and dysphagia. The client may complain of a "tight collar" sensation.   **(M-S)**

▶ When communicating with a client who has had a stroke, speak slowly, use visual cuing, face the client, use gestures, and repeat the information as necessary. **(M-S)**

▶ Any stress (for example, biological, environmental, psychological) can precipitate a sickle cell crisis. **(M-S)**

▶ An adolescent with diabetes insipidus should be taught to self-administer I.M. injections of vasopressin and to have nasal spray available for emergencies. **(PED)**

▶ Suspect coarctation of the aorta in a child with bounding pulses in the arms caused by the narrowing or constriction of the descending aorta. **(PED)**

▶ The most prevalent sexually transmitted disease in the United States is caused by *Chlamydia*. **(M-S)**

▶ Complications of prolonged, uncontrolled inflammation of asthma are lung remodeling and permanent changes in lung function. **(M-S)**

▶ Involve clients with bipolar disorder in activities that use the larger muscle groups and require less concentration, for example, ping-pong rather than checkers. **(PSY)**

▶ Signs of relapse of a polydrug user are visiting "old buddies," frequenting places where drugs or alcohol are sold or consumed, and skipping meals. **(PSY)**

▶ If a client requires more frequent administration of albuterol, the physician should be notified so the dose can be adjusted. **(M-S)**

▶ Toddlers are at the greatest risk for injury because they have increased mobility, curiosity, and ability to open containers, but lack the ability to properly assess dangers. **(PED)**

▶ Blood pressure should be monitored in a client with glomerulonephritis because of the associated sign of hypertension. **(M-S)**

▶ A male client who's quadriplegic can achieve an erection through stimulation of the genitalia because it's a reflex reaction. **(M-S)**

▶ Determining a client's cultural practices in order to meet his needs and preferences and provide culturally based care is called *cultural competence*. **(FND)**

▶ Changing to compensate for an existing condition is called *adaptation*. **(FND)**

▶ A lack of concern for one's own welfare in favor of another's health and welfare is called *altruism*. **(FND)**

▶ Assigning a task to a lower level trained nurse is called *delegation*. **(FND)**

▶ Assigning a task to an equally trained nurse is called *transfer of assignment*. **(FND)**

▶ Analyzing a situation and using available knowledge to deduce a reason or a decision is called *critical thinking*. **(FND)**

▶ *Empowerment* is the process of sharing power and is based on the assumption that people are capable and reasonable and can be trusted with decision making. **(FND)**

▶ If the client asks the nurse multiple questions about an upcoming surgery, assume that the client isn't informed and contact the physician. **(M-S)**

▶ *Transcultural nursing* refers to a review or study of various cultures and the care provided to clients relative to their view, values, and beliefs. **(FND)**

▶ When answering questions on the NCLEX, use the axiom "assess before action." This should prevent selecting an answer that's written in the "implementation" phase when a proper course would be "assessment." **(FND)**

▶ When reading a client-oriented question on the NCLEX, identify the goal for the particular client and then select the answer from the choices provided that meets or helps reach the goal. **(FND)**

▶ A nurse should accept only written "no code" orders from a physician. **(FND)**

▶ Hives are a sign of anaphylaxis in a client who has received a contrast medium for an intravenous pyelogram (IVP). Notify the physician immediately. **(M-S)**

▶ In clients with gouty arthritis, encourage the intake of large amounts of fluid (2,500 to 3,000 ml) to prevent the precipitation of urate in the kidneys. **(M-S)**

▶ The client with epididymitis will experience relief when the scrotum is placed on a pillow or other raised surface such as a towel. The client will feel a dragging sensation when ambulating; he should be advised to wear a scrotal support. **(M-S)**

▶ *Validation* is the process of double checking (for example, retaking an unusually high temperature before recording it and making other treatment decisions). **(FND)**

▶ Torsion testicle is a medical emergency usually requiring surgery. Essentially blood supply to the testicle is compromised. Failure to relieve compression will result in death to the tissue of the testicle. **(M-S)**

▶ Ambulating a client shortly after appendectomy decreases the risk of atelectasis and promotes the return of bowel sounds. **(M-S)**

▶ Signs and symptoms of renal hemorrhage in a client are pain and hematoma in the flank on the affected side. **(M-S)**

▶ A symptom of a duodenal ulcer is epigastric pain, which may be relieved by food. **(M-S)**

▶ The nurse can best protect herself against contamination when irrigating a wound by wearing a face shield, a mask, a gown, and gloves. **(FND)**

▶ Encourage a client with a urinary tract infection to drink cranberry juice. **(M-S)**

▶ Gonorrhea can cause irreparable damage to fallopian tubes, resulting in obstruction, increased risk of a tubal pregnancy, or sterility. **(MAT)**

▶ Compartment syndrome results from an accumulation of fluid within a muscle compartment, which decreases blood flow to tissues and can lead to neuromuscular deficiency and tissue death. **(M-S)**

▶ A client taking an anticholinesterase drug (for example, Mestinon) for myasthenia gravis should be told to take the medication 30 minutes before meals. **(M-S)**

▶ A client taking ColBenemid should be told to avoid an acid-ash diet. **(M-S)**

▶ Otosclerosis manifests as slow, progressive hearing loss. **(M-S)**

▶ Signs and symptoms of shigellosis are fever and crampy abdominal pain. In severe cases, the client may have bloody diarrhea and may need to be hospitalized for fluid support and other care. **(M-S)**

▶ A child with HIV-positive blood should receive inactivated poliovirus vaccine (IPV) immunization rather than oral poliovirus vaccine (OPV). **(PED)**

▶ A client with a hiatal hernia (esophageal hernia) should be instructed to remain in an upright position after eating. **(M-S)**

▶ Tympanic and skin thermometers are preferred for taking the temperature of an infant. **(PED)**

▶ The carotid pulse should only be taken on one side at a time to minimize the risk of obstructing blood flow to the brain. **(FND)**

▶ When taking a blood pressure reading, the cuff should be at the level of the heart. If it's above or below the heart, the blood pressure reading may be inaccurate. **(FND)**

▶ The purpose of catching the urine "midstream" is to prevent contamination by the labia (which should be separated during urination) or the opening of the urethra of the penis. **(FND)**

▶ A woman should have a mammogram annually starting at age 40. **(FND)**

▶ Common sites for intradermal injections are the inner arm, upper chest, and on the back beneath the scapula. **(FND)**

▶ A client will have less pain during an injection if the skin is pulled taut. **(FND)**

▶ The site where heparin or iron has been injected shouldn't be massaged.
(FND)

▶ Carbon monoxide is odorless, colorless, and tasteless; when inhaled, it can cause a range of symptoms, such as headache, dizziness, nausea, and even death. **(M-S)**

▶ Measures that can reduce a person's susceptibility to infection include good hygiene, proper nutrition, adequate rest, enough fluid, and lessened exposure (for example, limiting visits to health care clinics). **(FND)**

▶ Sterilization kills all microorganisms, including spores. **(FND)**

▶ If a client refuses to use an adaptive device, such as a hearing aid, assist the client to adapt without the device. **(FND)**

▶ By 3 years of age, a toddler usually demonstrates day-and-night bowel and bladder training. **(PED)**

▶ To ensure adequate nutrition of a hospitalized toddler, ask the parents about the child's specific dietary habits and food preferences. **(PED)**

▶ The developmental task of an adolescent is identity versus role confusion.
(PED)

▶ Breast development is a secondary sexual characteristic. **(PED)**

▶ Puberty is the period during which sexual organs begin to grow and mature.
(PED)

▶ Signs of shaken baby syndrome include seizures, slow apical pulse, difficulty breathing, and retinal hemorrhage. **(PED)**

▶ The leading cause of death of young adults is motor vehicle accidents.
(PED)

▶ A client is at greatest risk for infection during the 2 weeks following chemotherapy. **(M-S)**

▶ To reduce the risk of infection in a client with a vancomycin-resistant infection, contact precautions as well as standard precautions should be implemented.
(M-S)

▶ An incapacitated client's hair should be brushed or combed at least once daily.
(FND)

▶ When providing eye care for a comatose client, clean the eyes with saline solution, wiping from the inner to the outer canthus. **(FND)**

▶ The clinical test hemoglobin A_{1c} provides useful information on how well diabetes is being controlled. **(M-S)**

▶ The acid-fast bacillus (AFB) test requires that a sputum specimen be collected on 3 consecutive days. **(M-S)**

▶ If a client will have urine collected over a 24-hour period, post signs in the client's room, bathroom, and on the Kardex. **(FND)**

▶ A complete drug order contains the inclusive dates of administration, the client's name, the name of the drug, the amount of drug, time of administration (including PRN), and the name of the physician writing the order. **(FND)**

▶ When mixing one medication in an ampule and one in a multidose vial, draw the medication from the vial first. **(FND)**

▶ An emaciated client has an increased risk of pressure ulcers. **(FND)**

▶ Tepid water is between 80° and 98° F (26.6° and 36.6° C). **(FND)**

▶ Because of limited blood supply to adipose tissue, an obese client may experience difficulty with wound healing. **(M-S)**

▶ After placing a postoperative client in a bedside chair, caution him against slouching or crossing his legs. **(M-S)**

▶ The most serious mobility problem for an elderly client in the hospital is falls. **(FND)**

▶ When helping a client move up in bed, let the client use his own rocking motion to propel upward. **(FND)**

▶ A major risk for a nurse at work is back injury. **(FND)**

▶ The best position for a back rub is prone. **(FND)**

▶ Isometric exercises don't increase muscle mass but do maintain strength. **(FND)**

▶ Regarding the safe transportation of a client in a wheelchair, back the wheelchair in and out of elevators, make sure the client sits back in the seat and doesn't lean forward, and make sure that foot rests are down and the client's feet are resting on them. **(FND)**

▶ A treatment for intractable pain (pain that's resistant to cure) is a nerve block. **(M-S)**

▶ Expect the family to perform ritual cleaning and preparation of the body for a Muslim client who has died. **(FND)**

▶ The family of a deceased client may remain with the body for 2 to 3 hours, or before rigor mortis. **(FND)**

▶ A factor that may impair communication is failing to listen. **(FND)**

▶ The nurse should wear gloves when shaving a client with a safety razor. **(FND)**

▶ A whistling sound being emitted from a hearing aid indicates that it's turned up too loud. **(FND)**

▶ When a closed water-seal chest drainage system is attached properly to suction, fluctuation occurs in the water-seal chamber.   (M-S)

▶ During a liver biopsy, the nurse should instruct the client to hold his breath, turn his head to the left, and place his right hand under his head while the needle is inserted.   (M-S)

▶ After a liver biopsy, the nurse should position the client on his right side with a pillow under the liver border to place pressure on the puncture site.   (M-S)

▶ After a pneumonectomy, the nurse promotes full expansion of the client's unaffected lung by helping him ambulate, perform incentive spirometry, and lie on the affected side.   (M-S)

▶ When collecting a 24-hour urine specimen, the nurse should discard the first voiding, start the clock, and begin the 24-hour collection with the next specimen and the clock still running.   (M-S)

▶ The frequency of labor contractions is assessed by timing from the beginning of one contraction to the beginning of the next, and is measured in minutes.   (MAT)

▶ The duration of labor contractions is assessed by timing from the start to the end of the uterine muscle contraction, and is measured in seconds.   (MAT)

▶ For a client with epiglottiditis, the nurse should keep a tracheostomy set at the bedside for immediate use in case of airway obstruction.   (M-S)

▶ Spills of blood should be cleaned with a fresh 1:10 solution of sodium hypochlorite (household bleach) in water.   (M-S)

▶ If a child has recurrent otitis media, the nurse should question the parents about compliance with prescribed drug therapy.   (PED)

▶ To prevent hip flexion contractures after a leg amputation, the nurse should avoid placing the residual limb on pillows after the first 24 hours and elevating the head of the bed higher than 60 degrees. The client should be placed in a prone position twice daily.   (M-S)

▶ *Ritualistic behavior* is any repetitive act performed by a client who has obsessive-compulsive disorder.   (PSY)

▶ The best method to prevent nosocomial infections is hand washing after every client contact.   (M-S)

▶ A client with an amputation may have phantom sensation or pain. Pain is treated; sensation isn't.   (M-S)

▶ The nurse can acquire a nosocomial infection while performing usual nursing duties by not washing her hands after each direct or indirect client contact.   (M-S)

▶ After the nurse has contact with a client who's considered uncontaminated, hand washing for 15 to 30 seconds is considered sufficient for infection control. **(FND)**

▶ Mannitol (Osmitrol), a hypertonic solution, is used to treat clients with cerebral edema. **(M-S)**

▶ During therapy with mannitol or any I.V. diuretic, the client should have an indwelling urinary catheter so that urine output can be monitored accurately. **(M-S)**

▶ Rocky Mountain spotted fever is transmitted through the bite of a wood tick in the west and a dog tick in the east. **(M-S)**

▶ If a child is suspected of having epiglottiditis or croup, the nurse shouldn't examine the inside of the throat or even take an oral temperature. **(PED)**

▶ A characteristic sign of Lyme disease is an expanding bull's eye erythematous lesion that may appear anywhere on the body, at the site of the tick bite. **(M-S)**

▶ Giardiasis is an infection of the small bowel, caused by the symmetrical flagellate protozoan *Giardia lamblia*. Symptoms include diarrhea; abdominal cramps; and pale, loose, greasy, malodorous, and frequent stools. **(M-S)**

▶ A traction rope that has slipped out of the pulley should be placed back in the groove by a physician or registered nurse. **(M-S)**

▶ Round or cylindrical foods (such as raw carrots) shouldn't be given to a toddler because of the risk of aspiration. **(PED)**

▶ The organization that formulates nursing diagnoses is the North American Nursing Diagnosis Association (NANDA). **(FND)**

▶ Signs of *fetal alcohol syndrome* usually occur within the first 24 hours of life. **(PED)**

▶ One of the most common adverse GI effects of digoxin is nausea. **(M-S)**

▶ After circumcision, the infant should be closely monitored for bleeding. **(MAT)**

▶ Cervical dilation occurs in an inevitable abortion, but not in a threatened abortion. **(MAT)**

▶ Two medications used to treat Parkinson's disease are levodopa (Dopar) and carbidopa-levodopa (Sinemet). **(M-S)**

▶ Five types of hallucinations occur: visual, auditory, tactile, gustatory, and olfactory. **(PSY)**

▶ For the client who has a Sengstaken-Blakemore tube, the nurse should keep a pair of scissors at the bedside for cutting the tube for emergency deflation. **(M-S)**

▶ The fat-soluble vitamins are A, D, E, and K. (M-S)

▶ Starch is the most abundant dietary carbohydrate. (M-S)

▶ The nurse should assess for dependent edema in the lower extremities, such as the ankles (in a dependent position) in the ambulatory client or the sacrum in the wheelchair- or bed-bound client. (M-S)

▶ In an *autograft*, the client's own skin is taken from a donor site and transplanted to the graft site. (M-S)

▶ In a *homograft*, skin is taken from a cadaver 6 to 24 hours after death and transplanted to an individual of the same species. (M-S)

▶ The characteristic sign of primary syphilis is a painless, fluid-filled lesion (chancre) that can become painful if infected. (M-S)

▶ Many women who have the sexually transmitted disease gonorrhea have no signs or symptoms. (M-S)

▶ Ménière's disease causes a triad of symptoms: vertigo, hearing loss, and tinnitus. (M-S)

▶ Vitamin C promotes wound healing. It is found in brightly colored fruits and vegetables. (M-S)

▶ To decrease the risk of urinary tract infection, the client should wash the perineal area from front to back with soap and water twice daily and after each bowel movement. (M-S)

▶ A smooth, sore, red, beefy tongue (called *glossitis*) is a sign of pernicious anemia. (M-S)

▶ A major concern for the client receiving total parenteral nutrition is the risk of hyperglycemia. During treatment, the client will receive insulin on a sliding scale as needed. (M-S)

▶ To prevent hypoglycemia when total parenteral nutrition is being stopped, the nurse should gradually taper the amount administered, as ordered, and give the client oral carbohydrates. These actions allow the body to adjust to the decreasing glucose level. (M-S)

▶ To administer a routine enema effectively, the nurse should place the adult client on his left side. (M-S)

▶ The normal pH of arterial blood is 7.35 to 7.45. (FND)

▶ Split-thickness grafts, which include two upper layers of skin (epidermis) and part of the middle layer (dermis), are commonly used in early stages of burns. (M-S)

▶ In skin grafts, a heat lamp is used to dry the donor site, promote epithelization from deeper layers of skin, and prevent infection. (M-S)

▶ During heparin (Liquaemin) therapy, the client should receive acetaminophen (Tylenol), not aspirin, for headaches or other common pain complaints.
(M-S)

▶ In a small child or infant, the preferred site for I.M. injection is the vastus lateralis muscle. (FND)

▶ When trying to understand how a client feels about a disturbing issue, the nurse uses empathy, not sympathy. Sympathy is feeling sorry for another; empathy is understanding another's feelings. (PSY)

▶ Signs of lithium carbonate toxicity include diarrhea, vomiting, drowsiness, muscle weakness, and ataxia. (PSY)

▶ A milliequivalent (mEq) is the unit of measurement used to describe the chemical activity of electrolytes; mEq is the number of milligrams per 100 milliliters of a solution. (FND)

▶ When a client checks out of the hospital against a physician's advice, documentation should indicate that the client left AMA (against medical advice) and should include any significant reasons the client gave for leaving. (FND)

▶ Dietary fiber can't be digested by human enzymes and can't be absorbed from the small intestine. (M-S)

▶ A client who's immobilized should be provided with a footboard to prevent dorsiflexion of the foot and footdrop. (M-S)

▶ In chronic venous insufficiency, over time, collateral blood flow develops to the affected area. (M-S)

▶ In acute venous insufficiency, collateral blood flow doesn't have an opportunity to develop before tissue is damaged. (M-S)

▶ Motor impulses usually return 2 to 14 days after a stroke. (M-S)

▶ Oxytocin (Pitocin) is administered to promote uterine contractions. (MAT)

▶ During the latent phase of the first stage of labor, the client's cervix dilates from 0 to 4 cm. (MAT)

▶ During the active phase of the first stage of labor, the client's cervix dilates from 4 to 8 cm. (MAT)

▶ During the transitional phase of the first stage of labor, the client's cervix dilates from 8 to 10 cm. (MAT)

▶ During the first stage of labor, effacement becomes complete and expulsion of the neonate begins. (MAT)

▶ The second stage of labor begins with complete cervical effacement and dilation and ends with delivery of the fetus. (MAT)

▶ The third stage of labor begins after the birth of the neonate and ends with delivery of the placenta. **(MAT)**

▶ The fourth stage of labor begins with expulsion of the placenta and ends with postpartum stabilization. **(MAT)**

▶ *Pulse pressure* is the difference between the systolic and diastolic pressures. For example, if blood pressure is 120/80, pulse pressure is 40 mm Hg. **(M-S)**

▶ *Pulse deficit* is the difference between the apical pulse and a peripheral pulse such as the radial pulse. **(FND)**

▶ The nurse should weigh the client at the same time every day, using the same scale and with the client wearing the same type of clothing. **(FND)**

▶ If the client has cramping during colostomy irrigation, the nurse should lower the bag to slow the flow rate. **(M-S)**

▶ The nurse should turn the neonate often during phototherapy and keep him hydrated. **(MAT)**

▶ The three phases of a uterine contraction are increment, acme, and decrement. **(MAT)**

▶ Fever and chills are the most common transfusion reactions. **(M-S)**

▶ If jaundice is suspected in a neonate, the nurse should examine him under natural light or a white fluorescent light. **(MAT)**

▶ If a bottle-fed neonate doesn't begin to suck, the nurse should show the mother how to elicit the rooting reflex. **(MAT)**

▶ The first sign of bladder cancer is usually painless hematuria. **(M-S)**

▶ Before engaging in strenuous activity, a client with angina pectoris should take a nitroglycerin (Nitro-Bid) tablet. **(M-S)**

▶ A client with pernicious anemia must take vitamin B_{12} injections for the rest of his life. **(M-S)**

▶ The stress of hospitalization can precipitate a sickle cell crisis. **(M-S)**

▶ Maternal stress can decrease the breast milk supply. **(MAT)**

▶ Before administering an iron dextran (InFeD) injection, the nurse should change the needle on the syringe. **(M-S)**

▶ To prevent tooth staining, the child should use a straw to drink a liquid iron preparation. **(PED)**

▶ Annual rectal examinations aid in early detection of prostate cancer. **(M-S)**

▶ A sign of breast cancer is a nontender, nonmovable lump (usually in the upper outer quadrant). **(M-S)**

▶ A client with orthopnea must sit or stand to breathe deeply or comfortably. (M-S)

▶ A positive Homans' sign (calf pain on dorsiflexion of the foot) is a sign of deep vein thrombosis. (M-S)

▶ Before administering protamine sulfate as an antidote for heparin overdose, the nurse should verify that the client doesn't have an allergy to fish. (M-S)

▶ *Independent nursing actions* are actions that the nurse initiates, without direction from a physician, and has the requisite skills and knowledge to perform. (FND)

▶ *Subjective data* consist of information supplied by the client, a family member, or another health care provider that's based on opinion. (FND)

▶ *Objective data* consist of information that's observable or measurable. (FND)

▶ During the first 8 weeks after conception (the period of organogenesis), all organs are developed in a rudimentary form and the fetus is highly susceptible to a teratogenic effect. (MAT)

▶ Signs of inflammation include pain, erythema, swelling, warmth, and loss of motor function. (M-S)

▶ A *circadian rhythm* is a cycle that repeats about once daily (every 24 hours). (FND)

▶ When performing passive range-of-motion exercises, the nurse shouldn't force the extremity beyond the point of pain or continuous spasm. (FND)

▶ When shaving a client, the nurse should hold the razor at a 45-degree angle, use firm strokes, and follow the direction of hair growth. (FND)

▶ A slip knot is the best knot to use when securing a limb restraint because it's easy to release in case of emergency. (FND)

▶ The nurse should place a crib net over the crib to prevent a child younger than age 2 from climbing out. A child older than age 2 shouldn't be in a crib. (PED)

▶ A pregnant teenager should be encouraged to select foods that are high in iron and protein. (MAT)

▶ Clients with heart failure should avoid canned or processed foods, which are high in sodium. (M-S)

▶ A client who has Laënnec's cirrhosis should take vitamin B and fat-soluble vitamins (A, D, E, and K). (M-S)

▶ In a direct interview, the scope of discussion is confined, and the client is asked only specific questions. (FND)

▶ During furosemide (Lasix) therapy, the client is at risk for potassium loss, which can lead to hypokalemia. **(M-S)**

▶ Before obtaining a throat culture, the nurse should ask the client to rinse his mouth with water. **(M-S)**

▶ Before providing a sputum sample, the client shouldn't brush his teeth or use mouthwash. **(M-S)**

▶ Food eaten by an Orthodox Jewish client must be kosher. **(FND)**

▶ A sign of fecal impaction is seepage of liquid stool. **(M-S)**

▶ The feces of a breast-fed infant are golden yellow, smooth, and pasty. **(PED)**

▶ Meconium is thick and usually green to black. **(MAT)**

▶ In a dark-skinned client, the nurse should assess for petechiae on the oral mucosa rather than on the skin. **(M-S)**

▶ A woman who has Rh-negative blood should receive an injection of $Rh_o(D)$ immune globulin (RhoGAM) within 72 hours after giving birth to a neonate with Rh-positive blood. **(MAT)**

▶ Immediately after birth, the neonate's mouth and then nose should be suctioned. **(MAT)**

▶ When suctioning a tracheostomy, the nurse should apply suction as the catheter is withdrawn from the trachea and should limit the number of passes into and out of the trachea to two. **(M-S)**

▶ A client can hyperventilate by breathing too quickly or by breathing too deeply at a normal rate. **(M-S)**

▶ A client can hypoventilate by breathing too slowly or by breathing too shallowly at a normal rate. **(M-S)**

▶ The treatment for hypoventilation is controlled breathing or breathing into a paper bag. **(M-S)**

▶ For the mother who plans to breast-feed, the nurse should instruct her to "toughen" her nipples by rolling them between her thumb and forefinger or rubbing them with a towel. **(MAT)**

▶ A mother who plans to breast-feed should be permitted to do so shortly after delivery. **(MAT)**

▶ A probable sign of pregnancy is a positive human chorionic gonadotropin value in blood or urine. **(MAT)**

▶ Positive signs of pregnancy include fetal presence on ultrasound, palpable fetal movement, and fetal heart tones. **(MAT)**

▶ Presumptive signs of pregnancy include nausea, vomiting, and breast tenderness. **(MAT)**

▶ *Gravidity* is the total number of times that a woman has been pregnant, regardless of the outcome of the pregnancy. (MAT)

▶ *Parity* is the number of pregnancies that reached viability (20 weeks' gestation), regardless of whether the fetus was born alive. (MAT)

▶ For a 5-year-old child, one of the greatest fears about being hospitalized is the fear of mutilation. (PED)

▶ Weight gain after peritoneal dialysis indicates fluid retention and should be reported immediately to the unit manager. (M-S)

▶ Theophylline toxicity occurs when the serum theophylline level rises to greater than 20 mcg/ml. (M-S)

▶ Battered-child syndrome is one of the leading causes of childhood death and disability. (PED)

▶ When administering an antacid with cimetidine (Tagamet), the nurse should give the antacid 1 hour before the cimetidine. (M-S)

▶ After collecting a stool sample for ova and parasite testing, the nurse should send the sample immediately (while warm) to the laboratory. (M-S)

▶ A wound that heals with granulation is healing by secondary intention. (M-S)

▶ An ominous sign of increased intracranial pressure is widening pulse pressure. (M-S)

▶ A clinical sign of placenta previa is painless vaginal bleeding. (MAT)

▶ Fat provides 9 cal/g. (FND)

▶ Biological death occurs with the irreversible destruction and death of brain tissue. (FND)

▶ The nurse should use sterile technique when administering an I.M. injection. (FND)

▶ Range-of-motion (ROM) exercises should be performed on an immobilized client at least twice daily. (FND)

▶ *Active ROM exercises* are performed by the client. (FND)

▶ *Passive ROM exercises* are performed on the client by another individual. (FND)

▶ When performing ROM exercises, the nurse should stop the exercise based on her assessment of the client's previous level of tolerance. (FND)

▶ Respiratory insufficiency is the most common complication after pneumonectomy. (M-S)

▶ When wearing gloves, cuffs should be brought over gown sleeves. (FND)

▶ Medicare is a government-funded program that provides medical and hospital insurance to people age 65 and older.   **(FND)**

▶ In Freud's phallic stage, boys develop an Oedipus complex and girls develop an Electra complex.   **(PSY)**

▶ If liquid passes through a porous sterile field, the field is no longer considered sterile.   **(M-S)**

▶ *Sordes* is the accumulation of mucus and formation of crust on the teeth and lips.   **(M-S)**

▶ A client who's in a cast can maintain muscle mass and strength by performing isometric exercises.   **(FND)**

▶ According to Maslow's hierarchy of needs, physiologic needs must be met before other needs can be addressed.   **(FND)**

▶ During evaluation, the nurse determines whether the client's goals have been met.   **(FND)**

▶ *Linea nigra* is a dark line that runs from the umbilicus to the mons pubis during pregnancy.   **(MAT)**

▶ Implantation of the ovum occurs 7 to 10 days after fertilization.   **(MAT)**

▶ For the first 24 hours after leg amputation, the foot of the bed is raised to elevate the stump and prevent edema.   **(M-S)**

▶ Lung cancer is the leading cause of cancer-related deaths among men in the United States.   **(M-S)**

▶ Level of consciousness deteriorates in this order: alertness, lethargy, stupor, light coma, and deep coma.   **(M-S)**

▶ Parkinson's disease is a progressive neurologic disease.   **(M-S)**

▶ Generalized tonic-clonic seizures involve both hemispheres of the brain and cause both sides of the body to react.   **(M-S)**

▶ Generalized tonic-clonic seizures are usually preceded by an aura.   **(M-S)**

▶ Status epilepticus causes acute prolonged seizure activity with failure to regain consciousness between seizures.   **(M-S)**

▶ The ideal donor for a client who needs a kidney transplant is an identical twin.   **(M-S)**

▶ Lung cancer is the most common cancer in women in the United States.   **(M-S)**

▶ *Curling's ulcer* is a peptic or duodenal ulcer that's caused by severe stress associated with a serious burn.   **(M-S)**

▶ One way to determine and record blood loss after a hysterectomy is to count the number of perineal pads used; saturating one pad an hour or ten pads in 24 hours is considered hemorrhaging.   (MAT)

▶ The most common surgical treatment for benign prostatic hyperplasia is transurethral resection of the prostate.   (M-S)

▶ When a chest tube is attached to a drainage system, inhalation causes the water in the water-seal chamber to rise and exhalation causes it to fall.   (M-S)

▶ Spinal fusion is used to stabilize the spine.   (M-S)

▶ To logroll a client, the nurse can use a draw sheet or obtain help from one or more nurses.   (M-S)

▶ In placenta previa, abnormal implantation in the lower uterine segment causes the placenta to cover the internal cervical os partially or completely. (MAT)

▶ In central (total) placenta previa, the placenta completely covers the cervical os.   (MAT)

▶ In partial (incomplete) placenta previa, the placenta covers a portion of the cervical os.   (MAT)

▶ In marginal (lateral) placenta previa, the placenta covers one side of the cervical os.   (MAT)

▶ In abruptio placentae, a normally implanted placenta separates from the uterine wall prematurely.   (MAT)

▶ *Cutis marmorata* is a transient vasomotor response that occurs primarily in the extremities of infants who are exposed to cold.   (PED)

▶ *Eclampsia* is gestational hypertension.   (MAT)

▶ Mental retardation has four classifications: mild, moderate, severe, and profound.   (M-S)

▶ For the male client who has reached puberty, the major complication of mumps is orchitis, which can lead to sterility.   (M-S)

▶ In women, a common complication of gonorrhea is pelvic inflammatory disease.   (MAT)

▶ In Hirschsprung's disease (congenital megacolon), lack of peristalsis causes abdominal distention.   (M-S)

▶ *Scoliosis* is a lateral S-shaped spinal curvature.   (M-S)

▶ According to Freud, infants are in the oral stage of psychosexual development.   (PSY)

▶ The secondary stage of syphilis causes a rash on the palms and soles.   (M-S)

▶ Alcoholics Anonymous uses a 12-step program to achieve sobriety; however, an alcoholic is never considered cured. **(PSY)**

▶ For a client who's receiving total parenteral nutrition, the nurse should monitor glucose and electrolyte levels often and give insulin as needed and prescribed. **(M-S)**

▶ As many as 90% of substance abusers have relapses. **(PSY)**

▶ When taken together, alcohol and barbiturates have an additive effect that leads to severe depression of the central nervous system. **(M-S)**

▶ A lithium level of greater than 2 mEq/L is toxic. **(PSY)**

▶ A client who's taking a monoamine oxidase inhibitor should avoid tyramine-rich foods, such as aged cheese, chocolate, and monosodium glutamate.
(PSY)

▶ The nurse should use the bell of the stethoscope to hear low-pitched sounds such as heart murmurs. **(FND)**

▶ A severe complication of a fractured femur is excessive blood loss that can lead to shock and renal failure. **(M-S)**

▶ To prepare for peritoneal dialysis, a catheter is inserted through the abdominal wall and into the peritoneal space. **(M-S)**

▶ If more than 3 L of dialysate solution is returned during peritoneal dialysis, the nurse should notify the physician. **(M-S)**

▶ Hemodialysis removes nitrogenous wastes and excess water from the blood.
(M-S)

▶ During hemodialysis, wastes diffuse through a semipermeable membrane and into the dialysate. Water enters the dialysate by osmosis. **(M-S)**

▶ Kaposi's sarcoma is an opportunistic disease associated with acquired immunodeficiency syndrome. **(M-S)**

▶ Gangrene usually affects the digits first. **(M-S)**

▶ The nurse should use the diaphragm of the stethoscope to hear high-pitched sounds such as breath sounds. **(FND)**

▶ The blood pressure measurement commonly varies 5 to 10 mm Hg from one arm to the other; this difference is normal. **(FND)**

▶ The blood pressure cuff should cover about one-third of the client's upper arm. **(FND)**

▶ To assess blood pressure in an obese client, the nurse may need to use a thigh cuff and listen for heart sounds in the popliteal space. **(FND)**

▶ A blood pressure cuff that's too loose will yield a reading that's too high.
(FND)

▶ *Ptosis* is drooping of the eyelids.   (FND)

▶ Overflow incontinence is characterized by frequent loss of urine from the bladder.   (M-S)

▶ The nurse should perform a weight-bearing transfer only with a client who has at least one strong leg.   (FND)

▶ The first sign of a pressure ulcer is skin redness that blanches under pressure.   (M-S)

▶ A tilt table allows gradual movement from a horizontal to a vertical position.   (FND)

▶ Using a tilt table allows the client's body to compensate for position changes.   (FND)

▶ Sickle cell anemia involves a defect in hemoglobin.   (M-S)

▶ When measuring for crutches, the nurse should have the client wear the shoes that he will use for walking.   (FND)

▶ If a client has taken hormonal contraceptives exactly as prescribed, she should continue to take them, even if she misses her menstrual period.   (M-S)

▶ If a client misses two consecutive menstrual periods while taking hormonal contraceptives as prescribed, she should stop taking the pills, notify her physician, and have a pregnancy test.   (M-S)

▶ If a client misses taking one hormonal contraceptive tablet, she should take it as soon as she remembers (or should take two at the next scheduled interval) and continue with the usual schedule.   (M-S)

▶ If a client misses taking a hormonal contraceptive for two consecutive days, she should take two tablets each day for two days, resume the usual schedule, and use an additional contraceptive method for 1 week.   (M-S)

▶ Mechanical ventilation can maintain ventilation automatically for an extended time.   (M-S)

▶ Mechanical ventilation may be performed by a negative- or positive-pressure ventilator.   (M-S)

▶ Stable angina pectoris is characterized by substernal pain that's caused by myocardial ischemia and lasts 2 to 3 minutes.   (M-S)

▶ Angina that lasts for more than 20 minutes and isn't relieved by nitroglycerin indicates a developing myocardial infarction.   (M-S)

▶ The results of a nitroglycerin test are positive if nitroglycerin administration relieves angina.   (M-S)

▶ For a client with angina pectoris, the goal of treatment is to reduce the heart's workload.   (M-S)

▶ Nitroglycerin causes generalized vasodilation, which promotes blood flow to the heart muscle. (M-S)

▶ The nurse should teach a client who has angina and is receiving sublingual nitroglycerin (Nitro-Bid) to place a tablet under the tongue at the first sign of chest pain. (M-S)

▶ The client may repeat the nitroglycerin dosage every 5 to 15 minutes, for a maximum of three tablets. (M-S)

▶ If chest pain persists for longer than 15 minutes, the client should be instructed to go to the nearest health care facility. (M-S)

▶ Hemodialysis may be performed 24 hours before a kidney transplant to remove accumulated waste products from the blood. (M-S)

▶ After a radical mastectomy, the arm on the affected side may swell because the procedure removes lymph nodes and lymph vessels. (M-S)

▶ A client who has had a radical mastectomy shouldn't have blood drawn from the affected arm. (M-S)

▶ In placenta previa, bleeding is painless, is rarely fatal, and usually subsides spontaneously with the initial episode. (MAT)

▶ A client who has had a mastectomy is susceptible to lymphedema. (M-S)

▶ Usually, the treatment for abruptio placentae is immediate cesarean delivery. (MAT)

▶ Nurses should transport hospitalized infants or children in strollers, wheelchairs, or beds, but not in their arms. (M-S)

▶ When a protective device is used to restrain a client, the nurse should attach it to the bed frame or to springs that move with the client's head. (M-S)

▶ Signs of theophylline toxicity include vomiting, agitation, and an apical pulse of greater than 200 beats/minute. (M-S)

▶ When teaching the parents of a child with croup, the nurse should instruct them not to give cough syrup. (PED)

▶ The nurse shouldn't induce vomiting in a client who has ingested poison and is semiconscious, comatose, or experiencing seizures. (M-S)

▶ The nurse is required to report all suspected cases of child abuse to a child protective service agency. (PED)

▶ To prepare for a sigmoidoscopy, the nurse should place the client in the knee-chest or Sims' position. (M-S)

▶ The nurse should suspect sexual abuse in a child who has unexplained genital trauma or a sexually transmitted disease. (PED)

▶ *Central venous pressure* is the pressure in the right atrium and the great veins in the thorax.   (M-S)

▶ Central venous pressure normally is 2 to 8 mm Hg or 5 to 12 cm H_2O.   (M-S)

▶ Central venous pressure provides a guide for assessing right-sided cardiac function.   (M-S)

▶ Central venous access may be ordered to evaluate circulatory pressure in the right atrium and central veins.   (M-S)

▶ To administer subcutaneous heparin, the nurse should insert the needle into the skin at a 45-degree angle.   (FND)

▶ For the postoperative client who's at risk for deep vein thrombosis, heparin or enoxaparin (Lovenox) is usually given.   (M-S)

▶ Oral anticoagulants such as warfarin (Coumadin) prevent thrombus formation.   (M-S)

▶ Anticoagulants can't dissolve a thrombus that has already formed.   (M-S)

▶ Anticoagulant therapy is contraindicated in clients who have severe diabetes, liver or kidney disease, or ulcers.   (M-S)

▶ To assess a client for thrombophlebitis, the nurse should compare the measurements of the affected and unaffected limbs every day.   (M-S)

▶ Before moving the trauma client, the nurse should ensure that the airway is patent and that the cervical spine is immobilized.   (M-S)

▶ To prepare for sigmoidoscopy, the nurse should administer an enema 1 hour before the procedure.   (M-S)

▶ Administering a vasopressor, using ice water lavage, and inserting an esophageal balloon tamponade are treatments for bleeding esophageal varices.   (M-S)

▶ After a mastectomy, a symptom of lymphedema is a heavy sensation in the arm.   (M-S)

▶ It is appropriate for parents to tell their dying child that they will miss him.   (PED)

▶ A school-age child who's dying should be allowed to die while being comforted by family members.   (PED)

▶ An adolescent who's dying should be told the truth about his prognosis; however, the nurse should be careful to avoid presenting the situation as hopeless.   (PED)

▶ An adolescent who's dying may be resentful and may use denial as a defense mechanism.   (PED)

▶ When a dying client asks the nurse how much time he has left to live, she shouldn't provide an absolute time.   (M-S)

▶ After a child dies, the nurse should allow the family to spend time with the body. **(PED)**

▶ Usually, amniocentesis is performed at 12 to 16 weeks' gestation to detect inborn errors of metabolism. **(MAT)**

▶ A *sign* is an objective indication of a disease that can be perceived by an examiner. **(FND)**

▶ A *symptom* is a subjective indication of a disease or condition that's reported by the client. **(FND)**

▶ Many alcoholic individuals use alcohol to escape reality. **(PSY)**

▶ When a fracture is set in a child age 12 and younger, end-to-end apposition of the fractured ends isn't essential. **(PED)**

▶ Celiac disease is usually diagnosed at age 6 to 24 months. **(PED)**

▶ Treatment of celiac disease includes consumption of a gluten-free diet for the rest of the child's life. **(PED)**

▶ For the client with a disability, the ultimate nursing goal is to help the client reach his maximum health potential. **(FND)**

▶ Nitroglycerin tablets are considered expired 5 to 6 months after the bottle is opened. **(M-S)**

▶ Physiologic jaundice is common at the beginning of day 2 of life. It peaks at 1 week of life and disappears in the second week. **(MAT)**

▶ Pathologic jaundice is evident in the first 24 hours of life. **(MAT)**

▶ The puncture, or cutdown, site used for cardiac catheterization should be monitored for hematoma formation. **(M-S)**

▶ When using problem-oriented medical records, the health care team should focus on the client's problem list. **(FND)**

▶ *Myopia* is nearsightedness. **(FND)**

▶ *Hyperopia* is farsightedness. **(FND)**

▶ *Nystagmus* is rapid and involuntary horizontal, vertical, or rotating movement of the eyeballs. **(FND)**

▶ The optic disk is circular, appears yellowish-pink, and has a distinct border. **(FND)**

▶ When communicating with a child, the nurse should attempt to communicate at his eye level. **(PED)**

▶ The Weber test assesses hearing acuity through bone conduction. **(M-S)**

▶ The Rinne test evaluates hearing acuity by comparing air and bone conduction. **(M-S)**

▶ Signs of pacemaker failure include dizziness, fainting, palpitations, hiccups, and chest pain. (M-S)

▶ Primary disability results from a disease or disorder. (FND)

▶ When trying to elicit or clarify client information, the nurse should use open-ended questions. (FND)

▶ The failure rate of a birth control method is expressed as pregnancies per 100 women per year. (M-S)

▶ The *anteroposterior diameter* is the narrowest diameter of the pelvic inlet. (MAT)

▶ The *chorion* is the outermost embryonic membrane; it gives rise to the placenta. (MAT)

▶ The *amnion* is the innermost embryonic membrane. (MAT)

▶ The corpus luteum produces large quantities of progesterone. (MAT)

▶ The fetal period of development starts at the eighth week of gestation and continues until delivery. (MAT)

▶ Before the client with an amputation can be fitted for a prosthesis, the residual limb must be shrunk. (M-S)

▶ A client who has rheumatoid arthritis experiences the most severe pain starting in the small joints of the hands, wrists, and feet. (M-S)

▶ Autism usually first appears during infancy. (PED)

▶ In an incomplete abortion, the fetus is expelled, but parts of the placenta and amniotic membrane remain in the uterus. (MAT)

▶ Normally, a neonate has a head circumference of 13.8" (35 cm) and a chest circumference of 13" (33 cm). (MAT)

▶ During the first year, the infant's head and chest circumferences become equal. (PED)

▶ During the first period of reactivity, the neonate is alert, awake, and attentive. (MAT)

▶ A client who has placenta previa and vaginal bleeding should be placed in the semi-Fowler position. (MAT)

▶ Immediately after delivery, the highest priority is establishing a patent airway in the neonate. (MAT)

▶ Before getting the client out of bed for the first time after surgery, the nurse should have the client dangle his legs over the edge of the bed. (M-S)

▶ Greenstick fractures are the most common type of bone fractures in children. (PED)

▶ The nurse shouldn't induce vomiting in a client who has swallowed strychnine, hydrocarbon, or a strong acid or alkali. **(M-S)**

▶ Hydrocarbons can cause severe pneumonia if aspirated. **(M-S)**

▶ When placed under the tongue, nitroglycerin should cause a slight stinging sensation. **(M-S)**

▶ An infant with congenital hip dislocation has a positive Ortolani's sign. **(MAT)**

▶ A client who has cholecystitis may report clay-colored (pale) feces if the common bile duct is obstructed. **(M-S)**

▶ A pacemaker, surgical or orthopedic clips, or shrapnel will interfere with the results of a magnetic resonance imaging scan. **(M-S)**

▶ Benign prostatic hyperplasia typically causes urinary hesitancy and decreases the size and force of the urinary stream. **(M-S)**

▶ Distended jugular veins, ankle edema, and unexplained weight gain signal right-sided heart failure. **(M-S)**

▶ In a neonate, tremors or jitteriness may indicate hypoglycemia. **(MAT)**

▶ For neonates with opioid-induced respiratory depression at birth, naloxone (Narcan), an opioid antagonist, is the drug of choice. **(MAT)**

▶ Gestational hypertension usually resolves shortly after delivery. **(MAT)**

▶ Safety is a primary concern for a person who somnambulates (sleepwalks). **(M-S)**

▶ The optimal schedule for administering an around-the-clock antibiotic is 6 a.m., 12 p.m., 6 p.m., and 12 a.m. **(FND)**

▶ The nurse must follow standard precautions when caring for a client with hepatitis B. **(FND)**

▶ Clients who have obsessive-compulsive disorder can't control their behavior and receive no pleasure from it. **(PSY)**

▶ A woman should avoid pregnancy for 4 months after an abortion. **(MAT)**

▶ When opening a sterile surgical pack, the nurse should first open the top leaf of the protective towel away from herself. **(FND)**

▶ The nurse should adjust the fingers of sterile gloves only after putting on both gloves. **(FND)**

▶ The nurse should remove sterile gloves before removing a mask because the gloves are more contaminated than the mask. **(FND)**

▶ During a long sterile procedure, a mask that becomes moist should be covered with another sterile mask by someone who isn't in sterile attire. **(FND)**

▶ Activities of daily living include hygiene, elimination, environmental control, comfort measures, nutrition, activity, and mobility. (FND)

▶ After an endoscopy, the nurse should check the client for hemoptysis. (M-S)

▶ To determine a smoker's pack-year history, the nurse multiplies the number of packs smoked per day by the number of years that the person has been smoking. (FND)

▶ For a client who has eclampsia and is receiving magnesium sulfate, the nurse should assess for respiratory depression and diminished deep-tendon reflexes. (MAT)

▶ A diabetic client who becomes hypoglycemic should consume an easily digested carbohydrate, such as orange juice or a lump of sugar. (MAT)

▶ *Amino acids* are the end-product of protein digestion. (M-S)

▶ *Glycogenolysis* is the breakdown of glycogen into glucose. (M-S)

▶ Insulin is produced by the beta cells of the islets of Langerhans. (M-S)

▶ Glucagon is one of the hormones responsible for glycogenolysis. (M-S)

▶ Water-soluble vitamins aren't stored by the body. (M-S)

▶ *Oliguria* is the formation and excretion of less than 30 ml of urine an hour, or less than 500 ml during a 24-hour period. (FND)

▶ *Anuria* is the formation and excretion of less than 100 ml of urine in a 24-hour period. (FND)

▶ A client with Parkinson's disease should be instructed to walk with a broad-based gait (with feet apart). (M-S)

▶ The client with myasthenia gravis may have a sleepy, masklike facial expression. (M-S)

▶ For the client with myasthenia gravis who's receiving neostigmine methylsulfate (Prostigmin), the nurse should monitor for muscle weakness. (M-S)

▶ A client with myasthenia gravis who experiences diplopia should place an eye patch over one eye and move his head from side to side to enhance the visual field. (M-S)

▶ A client who has structural scoliosis should wear a Milwaukee brace 23 hours daily. (M-S)

▶ A client who has chronic pancreatitis requires pancreatic enzyme replacement and nutritional supplements. (M-S)

▶ The nurse should encourage the client who has diabetes to exercise regularly every day, usually starting the exercise 90 minutes after a meal. (M-S)

▶ A client who has a tracheostomy should humidify the air in his home. (M-S)

▶ The nurse should instruct the postmastectomy client to exercise the affected arm to prevent frozen shoulder and lymphedema. **(M-S)**

▶ A woman who has had a unilateral oophorectomy ovulates every other month. **(M-S)**

▶ Cancer spreads by invasion or by metastasis. **(M-S)**

▶ A client who has unstable angina experiences pain at rest. **(M-S)**

▶ A client who has a nihilistic delusion denies the reality or existence of the self, part of the self, or some external object. **(PSY)**

▶ To measure the amount of liquid medication in a medicine cup, the nurse holds the medicine cup at eye level and measures at the bottom of the meniscus. **(FND)**

▶ While administering a heparin injection, aspirating for blood return could cause a hematoma. **(M-S)**

▶ If a client has difficulty swallowing an oral medication, the nurse should advise him to place the medication as far back in his throat as possible. **(FND)**

▶ After administering a vaginal suppository, the nurse should instruct the client to remain supine for 5 to 10 minutes. **(FND)**

▶ When giving a Z-track injection, the nurse should use the dorsogluteal, ventrogluteal, or vastus lateralis site. **(FND)**

▶ Measles, mumps, and rubella immunization is usually given at age 12 to 15 months. **(PED)**

▶ Atelectasis typically occurs 24 to 48 hours after surgery. **(M-S)**

▶ During the first trimester of pregnancy, the woman should gain 3 to 5 lb (1.5 to 2.5 kg). **(MAT)**

▶ The adverse effects of vincristine (Oncovin) are alopecia, nausea, and vomiting. **(M-S)**

▶ For the client with hemiplegia, placing a pillow under the affected extremity encourages flexion deformity and impedes circulation. **(M-S)**

▶ When using a cane, the client should stand erect and carry the cane on the unaffected side. **(M-S)**

▶ When caring for the potentially suicidal client, ensuring client safety is the nurse's highest priority. **(PSY)**

▶ The most common adverse effect of electroconvulsive therapy is postshock amnesia. **(PSY)**

▶ A postoperative client who received general anesthesia is at risk for aspiration until he regains consciousness. The client should be positioned on his side or have his head turned to the side if side-lying positions are contraindicated.

(M-S)

▶ Atropine is given preoperatively to diminish secretions.   (M-S)

▶ The nurse should advise a client who has had an adverse drug reaction to withhold the next medication dose and call the physician immediately.   (FND)

▶ Cervical dilation occurs with true labor and is considered the primary difference between true and false labor.   (MAT)

▶ The nurse should assess fetal heart tones immediately after the amniotic membranes rupture.   (MAT)

▶ A client who's receiving epidural anesthesia during labor should be placed on her side, with her head slightly raised.   (MAT)

▶ In dark-skinned persons, skin color changes can best be seen in areas of less pigmentation, such as lips, mucous membranes, ear lobes, palms, and soles.

(M-S)

▶ Raisins are a good snack for a child who has iron deficiency anemia; eating vegetables every day is also recommended.   (PED)

▶ When working with a schizophrenic client, the nurse must gain the client's trust.   (PSY)

▶ Before removing a urinary catheter that has been in place for more than a few days, the nurse should clamp the catheter several times daily.   (M-S)

▶ A neonate who weighs 7 lb (3.2 kg) at birth should weigh 14 lb (6.4 kg) by age 6 months and 21 lb (9.5 kg) by age 12 months.   (MAT)

▶ A gluten-free diet allows rice, but excludes such foods as oats, wheat, and barley.   (M-S)

▶ Accidents are the leading cause of death in children ages 1 to 4.   (PED)

▶ A child who's playing alone with toys that differ from those used by nearby children is engaging in solitary play.   (PED)

▶ Parallel play is typically seen in toddlers who play independently, but alongside other children.   (PED)

▶ Tay-Sachs disease occurs primarily in Ashkenazi (eastern European) Jews and is manifested by cherry-red spots on the macula.   (M-S)

▶ Fraternal (dizygotic) twins derive from the fertilization of two separate ova.

(MAT)

▶ Identical (monozygotic) twins derive from the fertilization of one ovum.

(MAT)

▶ Monozygotic twins have an identical genetic makeup.   (MAT)

▶ Dizygotic twins have separate and distinct placentas and membranes. (MAT)

▶ A *fetal teratogen* is any agent or substance that can cause an adverse effect in a developing fetus.   (MAT)

▶ An infant's breathing is primarily abdominal.   (MAT)

▶ A rectal thermometer typically has a blunt, rounded bulb; an oral thermometer has a slender, elongated tip.   (FND)

▶ Marbling and speckling of the iris (Brushfield's spots) is seen in children with Down syndrome.   (PED)

▶ A female neonate may have pseudomenstruation.   (MAT)

▶ The normal umbilical cord consists of two arteries and one vein.   (MAT)

▶ Vitamin K is administered to neonates shortly after birth to prevent hemorrhage.   (MAT)

▶ A fractured clavicle (collarbone) is a common birth injury in large-for-gestational-age neonates.   (MAT)

▶ The therapeutic range of digoxin is 0.5 to 2 mg/ml.   (M-S)

▶ If a pregnant client becomes dizzy on the examination table, the nurse should place the client on her left side.   (MAT)

▶ Immediately after delivery, the neonate should be suctioned to ensure an adequate airway and normal breathing.   (MAT)

▶ The nurse should keep calcium gluconate 10% at the bedside of a client who's receiving magnesium sulfate for administration if signs of respiratory depression develop.   (M-S)

▶ Estriol determination is used to assess placental function and fetal well-being.   (MAT)

▶ If the fetus has a prolapsed umbilical cord, the nurse should place the mother in Trendelenburg's position or the knee-chest position, with the hips elevated.   (MAT)

▶ A variation from the normal fetal heart rate pattern may indicate fetal distress.   (MAT)

▶ Pelvic thrombophlebitis most commonly occurs about 2 weeks after delivery.   (M-S)

▶ The most common cause of postpartum hemorrhage is uterine atony. (MAT)

▶ Signs of tracheoesophageal fistula in the neonate include excessive nasal secretions, drooling, and violent choking during feeding.   (MAT)

▶ Respiratory distress syndrome is common in premature neonates.   (MAT)

► To reduce the risk of aspiration, the nurse should feed an infant who has a cleft lip or palate in an upright position.   (MAT)

► If water accumulates in the tubing of an oxygen delivery system, the nurse should disconnect the tubing and empty the water.   (M-S)

► Before administering morphine sulfate, the nurse should check the client's respiratory rate; if it's less than 12 breaths/minute, the nurse should withhold the drug and call the physician.   (M-S)

► As soon as surgery ends, a temporary drainage appliance is placed on a new ileostomy.   (M-S)

► Laboratory values that are elevated after a myocardial infarction include creatine kinase (CK), CK-MB, and lactate dehydrogenase-1.   (M-S)

► A child who's experiencing night terrors awakens screaming and can't recall what caused the frightening episode.   (PED)

► Narcolepsy is characterized by an uncontrollable desire to sleep.   (M-S)

► Bruxism is unconscious grinding or clenching of the teeth, especially during sleep.   (M-S)

► *Chronic pain* is limited, intermittent, or persistent pain of more than 6 months' duration.   (FND)

► *Acute pain* is transient pain of sudden onset, varying intensity, and less than 6 months' duration.   (FND)

► Signs and symptoms of acute myelogenous leukemia include increased susceptibility to infection, weakness, fatigue, bleeding, and enlarged lymph nodes.
                                                                             (M-S)

► In acute myelogenous leukemia, bleeding is caused by decreased platelet production.   (M-S)

► The nurse should avoid palpating the abdomen of a child who has Wilms' tumor because palpation could cause metastasis.   (PED)

► A client who's taking anticoagulants as an outpatient should be instructed to call the physician if he has black, tarry feces.   (M-S)

► The nurse should reassure parents that breast engorgement is normal in neonates.   (MAT)

► The first deciduous teeth to erupt in an infant are the lower central incisors.
                                                                             (PED)

► The two major stages of sleep are non–rapid-eye-movement and rapid-eye-movement sleep.   (M-S)

► The neonate's posterior fontanel may not be visible at delivery because of molding; it usually closes by age 2 to 3 months.   (MAT)

▶ The mature ovum and sperm each contain 23 chromosomes.   (MAT)

▶ Sperm retain their fertilizing capability for at least 48 hours after sexual intercourse.   (MAT)

▶ The joint action of luteinizing hormone and follicle-stimulating hormone cause the ovarian follicle to mature.   (MAT)

▶ Women should perform breast self-examination at least every month, about 1 week after menses.   (M-S)

▶ Men should check their testicles for masses at least every month, preferably during or shortly after a warm shower or bath.   (M-S)

▶ Early signs of croup can be managed at home by placing the child in a bathroom, closing the door, and running hot water in the shower or bathtub to create steam to break up the mucus.   (PED)

▶ A low-calcium diet is prescribed for clients who are at increased risk for renal calculi (such as immobilized clients).   (M-S)

▶ One gram of protein contains 4 calories.   (FND)

▶ Vitamin K deficiency may affect blood coagulation.   (M-S)

▶ A post-prostatectomy client who's receiving estrogen may experience breast enlargement (gynecomastia).   (M-S)

▶ If a client who's on a respirator becomes restless, he may need suctioning.   (M-S)

▶ The body stores glucose as glycogen.   (M-S)

▶ Broccoli, cabbage, and collard greens are high in calcium.   (M-S)

▶ During the fight-or-flight response, the release of glucagon and epinephrine is responsible for the conversion of glycogen to glucose.   (PSY)

▶ To prevent rickets, a person must consume adequate amounts of calcium and vitamin D.   (M-S)

▶ For the client with chronic obstructive pulmonary disease, high oxygen levels inhibit the respiratory drive.   (M-S)

▶ A client who breathes out while the mechanical ventilator is on the inspiratory cycle is said to be "fighting" the ventilator.   (M-S)

▶ The nurse should monitor the partial thromboplastin time of the client who's receiving heparin.   (M-S)

▶ During the orientation phase of the therapeutic relationship, clients often display testing and resistive behavior.   (FND)

▶ Postmenopausal bleeding is a common sign of uterine cancer.   (M-S)

▶ The most common sign of laryngeal cancer is hoarseness or a change in the voice. **(M-S)**

▶ Pain that radiates to the left shoulder from the splenic region suggests splenic rupture. **(M-S)**

▶ To prevent plantar flexion in the bedridden client, the nurse should use a footboard or have the client wear high-top athletic shoes. **(M-S)**

▶ Nocturnal enuresis (involuntary urination during sleep) typically occurs during stage II of non–rapid-eye-movement sleep. **(M-S)**

▶ The nurse should instruct the client who has gout to avoid organ meats such as liver because of their high purine content. **(M-S)**

▶ A trochanter roll should extend from the crest of the ilium to the mid-thigh. **(M-S)**

▶ To determine whether a client has a pulse deficit, one nurse should measure the apical pulse while a second nurse measures the radial pulse at the same time, using the same watch. **(FND)**

▶ A client who has hypothyroidism can't tolerate cold. **(M-S)**

▶ A client who has hyperthyroidism can't tolerate heat. **(M-S)**

▶ The nurse should make sure that the client is dried thoroughly after a bath. **(FND)**

▶ When a toddler is hospitalized, the nurse should ask the parents about the child's sleep rituals and the words he uses to communicate. **(PED)**

▶ To help assess a client's judgment, the nurse should ask such questions as, "If you found a stamped, addressed envelope, what would you do with it?" or "If you saw a fire in a crowded theater, what would you do?" **(FND)**

▶ After a bone marrow aspiration, the nurse should apply pressure to the puncture site for 5 to 10 minutes to ensure hemostasis. **(M-S)**

▶ In an immunosuppressed client, the client's own microorganisms are the most common cause of infection. **(M-S)**

▶ After a cholecystectomy, a T tube is inserted into the common bile duct for about 10 days to allow drainage of bile. **(M-S)**

▶ Sharp pain in the right upper abdominal quadrant that radiates to the back or the right shoulder is a common symptom of cholecystitis. **(M-S)**

▶ Before a cholangiogram, the nurse should assess the client for allergies, especially to iodine or shellfish. **(M-S)**

▶ An oral cholangiogram is performed only if ultrasound is unavailable or yields inconclusive results. **(M-S)**

▶ A client who's scheduled for a cholecystogram should take oral dye tablets 2 to 3 hours after the evening meal on the night before the test, or 10 to 12 hours before the test.   (M-S)

▶ During I.V. cholangiography, I.V. radioactive isotopes are injected.   (M-S)

▶ Adverse reactions to contrast media range from nausea and vomiting to hives and anaphylactic shock.   (M-S)

▶ If Rocky Mountain spotted fever is suspected, the nurse should ask whether the client has been in the woods lately or has been bitten by a tick.   (M-S)

▶ Having the client say "ahhh" when obtaining a throat culture relaxes the throat muscles and diminishes the gag reflex.   (FND)

▶ The nurse should obtain a specimen for a wound culture from the wound drainage area.   (M-S)

▶ One tablespoon of liquid feces or 1" (2.5 cm) of formed stool is usually sufficient for laboratory analysis.   (FND)

▶ Normal vaginal or urethral discharge is minimal, clear or white, and contains no pus or blood.   (M-S)

▶ The nurse shouldn't withhold oral intake before an EEG because the resulting hypoglycemia may alter test results.   (M-S)

▶ Before an EEG, the client's hair and scalp should be shampooed.   (M-S)

▶ A client who has pernicious anemia commonly experiences hypochlorhydria or achlorhydria.   (M-S)

▶ Persistent obstruction of the portal venous circulation usually leads to esophageal varices.   (M-S)

▶ After an upper GI endoscopy, the client should receive nothing by mouth until the normal gag reflex returns.   (M-S)

▶ After an upper GI endoscopy, the client may have slightly bloody sputum if a tissue biopsy sample was obtained from an area high in the esophagus.
                                                                          (M-S)

▶ On the morning before an upper GI X-ray, the nurse should instruct the client not to smoke or chew gum because these actions stimulate gastric motility.
                                                                          (M-S)

▶ After an upper GI X-ray, the nurse should instruct the client to increase fluid intake and eat a high-fiber diet to promote the passage of barium.   (M-S)

▶ Glucose breaks down into carbon dioxide and water.   (M-S)

▶ The nurse should instruct a client with diabetes to check his blood glucose level before each meal and at bedtime.   (M-S)

▶ When performing a fingerstick blood glucose test, the nurse should blot away the first drop of blood because it may be diluted with body fluids.   (M-S)

▶ Before contrast medium is injected, the nurse should tell the client to expect a transient burning sensation and a metallic taste in his mouth.   (M-S)

▶ Normal cerebrospinal fluid is clear and colorless.   (M-S)

▶ After a lumbar puncture, the client should lie flat in bed for at least 8 hours.   (M-S)

▶ If the client's cerebrospinal fluid pressure rises after a lumbar puncture, the nurse should take the client's vital signs and perform a neurologic assessment every 15 minutes for the first 4 hours, then every hour for the next 2 hours.   (M-S)

▶ After cataract removal, the client should avoid bending over, coughing, sneezing, or engaging in any activity that increases intraocular pressure.   (M-S)

▶ After a myelogram followed by removal of a non–water-soluble agent, the client must be returned to the room on a stretcher and must lie flat.   (M-S)

▶ Before examining a child's ear, the nurse should clean it with a soft moist cloth.   (PED)

▶ When examining an adult's ear, the nurse should pull the auricle up and back to straighten the ear canal.   (M-S)

▶ After instillation of eardrops, the client should lie on the opposite side of treatment for 5 to 10 minutes.   (M-S)

▶ To prevent damage to the cornea, the nurse should instill eyedrops into the conjunctiva and apply ointment on the edge of the lower conjunctival sac. (M-S)

▶ Cancer can occur anywhere in the colon, but is most commonly found in the rectum and sigmoid colon.   (M-S)

▶ A change in bowel habits is the most common presenting sign of colon cancer.   (M-S)

▶ A client with ulcerative colitis should eat a low-residue, high-protein diet.   (M-S)

▶ Placing one hand on the throat is the universal sign of choking.   (M-S)

▶ The client's identification bracelet should stay in place until he leaves the hospital grounds.   (FND)

▶ The most reliable way to identify a client is to check his identification bracelet. All other ways are secondary.   (FND)

▶ The nurse should begin discharge planning when the client is admitted.   (FND)

▶ During the client's hospital orientation, the staff should demonstrate proper use of the call bell system. **(FND)**

▶ *Clonus* is the rapidly alternating, involuntary contraction and relaxation of muscles. **(M-S)**

▶ For the client who needs ambulatory assistive aids, the nurse should explain the procedure, assemble the necessary equipment, and then help the client ambulate. **(M-S)**

▶ Dangling the client's legs before getting him out of bed helps prevent pooling of blood and orthostatic hypotension. **(M-S)**

▶ A postoperative client should receive pain medication 30 minutes before ambulating. **(M-S)**

▶ If the client has weakness on one side of his body, the nurse should stand on the weak side to provide support during rising and ambulation. **(M-S)**

▶ The nurse should place the client's bed in the lowest position after giving a bed bath and performing other care activities and should then place the call button within reach. **(M-S)**

▶ A client with hemiplegia should have his position changed at least every 2 hours and should be placed mainly on the unaffected side, with only brief periods on the affected side. **(M-S)**

▶ Water for a bed bath should be heated to 110° to 115° F (43.3° to 46° C). **(FND)**

▶ A fiberglass cast dries immediately after application. **(M-S)**

▶ A therapeutic bath contains an additive, such as oatmeal, cornstarch, sodium bicarbonate, oil, or a medication. **(FND)**

▶ To avoid transmitting microorganisms, the nurse should avoid direct contact between her uniform and the client's bed linens. **(FND)**

▶ When moving a bedridden client, rolling the client toward the nurse reduces strain and exertion. **(M-S)**

▶ Until a plaster cast is completely dry, the nurse should handle it with her palms. **(M-S)**

▶ An extremity that has a plaster cast should be turned every 2 hours to promote even drying. **(M-S)**

▶ Cystitis, an inflammation of the urinary bladder, usually results from an infection that ascends from the urethra. **(M-S)**

▶ Candidiasis is a fungal infection caused by *Candida albicans*. **(M-S)**

▶ The nurse should tape the indwelling urinary catheter of a female client to the client's leg. **(M-S)**

▶ When inserting a urinary catheter in a male client, the nurse should raise the penis to an angle of 60 to 90 degrees. **(M-S)**

▶ The practical or vocational nurse should complete only the original copy of an incident report and then submit the report to a registered nurse. **(FND)**

▶ A pregnant client who has poor balance should take showers instead of baths. **(MAT)**

▶ Respiratory depression is a common adverse effect of morphine. **(M-S)**

▶ Macronutrients are essential nutrients that supply energy and build tissue; they include carbohydrates, fats, and proteins. **(M-S)**

▶ Green, leafy vegetables are good sources of magnesium and vitamin K. **(M-S)**

▶ *Metabolism* is the chemical change within the body that makes energy available. **(M-S)**

▶ If the client is using a handheld inhaler (nebulizer), the nurse should instruct him to wait 30 to 60 seconds after the first puff before taking a second puff. **(M-S)**

▶ To drain the apical sections of the upper lung lobes using postural drainage, the nurse should have the client sit in high Fowler's position. **(M-S)**

▶ On percussion, areas that contain air or gas produce tympany, a drumlike sound. **(FND)**

▶ Black or tarry feces are associated with upper GI bleeding or a diet high in red meat or dark green vegetables. **(M-S)**

▶ Before collecting a stool specimen, the nurse should instruct the client to urinate and to avoid placing toilet paper in the stool sample. **(M-S)**

▶ For best results, the client should retain an oil-retention enema for at least 30 minutes. **(M-S)**

▶ When obtaining a urine sample from an indwelling urinary catheter, the nurse should clamp the tubing, allow the urine to collect, and then insert a 21G to 25G 1" needle through an injection port. **(M-S)**

▶ The normal ratio of carbonic acids to bicarbonate ions is 1:20. **(M-S)**

▶ To measure the amount of urine in a diaper, the nurse should subtract the weight of a dry diaper from the weight of the wet diaper and convert the number of grams to milliliters (1 gram in weight = 1 milliliter in volume). The weight can be determined by placing a dry, same-size diaper on a protective barrier on the scale, balancing the scale to 0, removing the dry diaper, and replacing it with the wet diaper. **(PED)**

▶ The *anion gap* is the difference between the concentrations of serum anions and cations. It's determined by subtracting the sum of chloride and bicarbonate anions from sodium cations. **(M-S)**

▶ Microdrip I.V. tubing delivers 60 gtt/ml. (M-S)

▶ Macrodrip I.V. tubing delivers 10, 15, 20, or 30 gtt/ml, depending on the manufacturer. (M-S)

▶ Sodium is the major cation in extracellular fluid. (M-S)

▶ To prevent vomiting, postural drainage should be performed 1 to 2 hours after the client eats a meal. (M-S)

▶ *Tidal volume* is the amount of air inspired and expired in a normal respiration. (M-S)

▶ *Surfactant* is a mixture of lipoproteins in the lungs that reduces the surface tension of pulmonary fluids. (M-S)

▶ *Hemoglobin* is an oxygen-carrying pigment in red blood cells. (M-S)

▶ Kussmaul's respirations are a compensatory response to metabolic acidosis. (M-S)

▶ Abnormal breath sounds are called *adventitious*. (M-S)

▶ An incentive spirometer is sometimes called a *sustained maximal inspiration device*. (M-S)

▶ When teaching pursed-lip breathing, the nurse should instruct the client to inhale through the nose and then exhale slowly and evenly against pursed lips while tightening the abdominal muscles. (M-S)

▶ When instilling drops in the ear, press gently on the tragus to promote the flow of medication toward the eardrum. (M-S)

▶ Body fat contains a small amount of water, whereas lean tissue is rich in water. (M-S)

▶ Women have proportionally more body fat, and therefore less body fluid, than men. (M-S)

▶ *Sebum* is the fatty secretion of a sebaceous gland. (M-S)

▶ *Diffusion* is the movement of a solute from an area of higher concentration to an area of lower concentration. (M-S)

▶ *Osmosis* is the movement of water across a semipermeable membrane from a less concentrated solution to a more concentrated solution. (M-S)

▶ *Active transport* is the movement of a solute across a concentration gradient; it requires energy. (M-S)

▶ *Hydrostatic pressure* is the pressure exerted by a liquid against the walls of a container within a closed system. (M-S)

▶ Thoracic breathing is costal, whereas abdominal breathing is diaphragmatic. (M-S)

▶ Respiratory depth is described as normal, deep, or shallow. **(FND)**

▶ A normal inspiration lasts 1 to 1½ seconds; a normal expiration lasts 2 to 3 seconds. **(FND)**

▶ In a *pureed diet,* food is blended to a semisolid consistency. **(M-S)**

▶ A clear liquid diet provides fluid and electrolytes, but lacks adequate fats, proteins, vitamins, calories, and minerals. **(M-S)**

▶ Before feeding a client, the nurse should ask the client if he prefers to eat foods in any particular order. **(FND)**

▶ The typical large-bore nasogastric (NG) tube is a #12 to #14 French tube. **(FND)**

▶ The client who's at risk for aspiration should receive an intestinal tube rather than a gastric tube. **(M-S)**

▶ The nurse should check the placement of an NG tube every 4 to 6 hours and before any bolus feeding. **(M-S)**

▶ A large-bore NG tube is more likely than a small-bore NG tube to cause coughing or choking when it enters the respiratory tract. **(M-S)**

▶ Total body water accounts for approximately 75% of the neonate's weight. **(FND)**

▶ Dextrose 5% in water, lactated Ringer's solution, and normal saline solution are examples of isotonic solutions. **(FND)**

▶ Half-normal saline solution (0.45% sodium hydrochloride solution) is an example of a hypotonic solution. **(FND)**

▶ An example of a hypertonic solution is 50% glucose. **(FND)**

▶ Fluid loss is considered insensible when it isn't perceptible. Such loss includes fluid lost from the skin through evaporation and fluid lost from the lungs as moisture exhaled during respiration. **(FND)**

▶ *Chyme* is a semifluid material that's produced by the digestion of food in the stomach. **(FND)**

▶ The most common cause of pulmonary edema is left-sided heart failure. **(M-S)**

▶ Diuretic use is the leading cause of potassium deficit. **(M-S)**

▶ Potassium is the major cation in intracellular fluid. **(M-S)**

▶ The nurse should instruct a client with tuberculosis to cover his mouth with a tissue when he coughs and to dispose of used tissues as biological waste. **(M-S)**

▶ Signs of tension pneumothorax include rapid, shallow respirations, chest pain, and cyanosis. **(M-S)**

▶ An elderly client who becomes confused as night approaches may be experiencing sundowning syndrome. **(M-S)**

▶ A Denis Browne splint is used for a child with clubfoot. **(PED)**

▶ To be prepared to clamp a chest tube, the nurse should keep two rubber-tipped clamps available for immediate use. **(M-S)**

▶ The sinoatrial node is the heart's natural pacemaker. **(M-S)**

▶ The T wave represents repolarization of the ventricles. **(M-S)**

▶ To avoid exposure to bacteria during wound care, the nurse should wear clean gloves when removing the top dressing. **(M-S)**

▶ Functional nursing focuses on tasks and procedures. **(FND)**

▶ An autocratic leader assumes complete control over decisions involving the group. **(FND)**

▶ In the dark-skinned client, the nurse should check for jaundice by inspecting the hard palate. **(M-S)**

▶ Fat digestion occurs primarily in the small intestine. **(M-S)**

▶ Carbohydrate digestion begins in the mouth. **(M-S)**

▶ *Surgical asepsis* is the practice of keeping an area or object free of all microorganisms and spores. **(FND)**

▶ Metamucil should be mixed in water before it's swallowed. **(M-S)**

▶ For an infant, the nurse should check skin turgor above the umbilicus. **(PED)**

▶ Before applying antiembolism stockings, the nurse should have the client lie down for 20 minutes with his feet elevated. **(M-S)**

▶ *Osteoporosis* is a demineralization process in which bones become less dense. **(M-S)**

▶ Having the client ambulate is the best way to prevent osteoporosis. **(M-S)**

▶ To assess a client for dehydration, the nurse should check skin turgor. **(M-S)**

▶ Chest tubes should be removed if fluid drainage is less than 50 ml daily. **(M-S)**

▶ *Sleep apnea* is transient cessation of breathing during sleep. **(M-S)**

▶ Sleep apnea is commonly associated with snoring. **(M-S)**

▶ After a diagnostic study in which the femoral site is used, the client must lie flat for 8 hours. **(M-S)**

▶ When caring for a client who has undergone a cardiac catheterization, the nurse must report a rapid or irregular pulse immediately. **(M-S)**

▶ An immobilized client should eat a diet that's high in protein, calories, and fiber, with liberal amounts of fluid. **(M-S)**

▶ The best method to verify lung reexpansion is with a chest X-ray; other methods include auscultation and percussion. **(M-S)**

▶ A high alpha-fetoprotein level after the 15th week of gestation is associated with spinal cord defects. **(MAT)**

▶ *Autonomy* implies freedom, self-control, and the ability to make independent decisions. **(FND)**

▶ *Third spacing* is the shifting of body fluids into a space that normally doesn't contain fluid. **(M-S)**

▶ The characteristic pattern of Guillain-Barré syndrome is ascending weakness that starts in the lower extremities and spreads upward to the trunk, upper extremities, and face. Respiratory compromise is a concern. **(M-S)**

▶ *False imprisonment* is the unjustifiable retention or prevention of the client's movement without proper consent or authority. **(FND)**

▶ *Euthanasia* is the deliberate termination of a person's life when the person is suffering from a painful or fatal condition. **(FND)**

▶ A *living will* is a document that describes a client's wishes for treatment in the event that he becomes unable to communicate his wishes. **(FND)**

▶ A neonate should pass meconium 24 to 48 hours after birth. **(MAT)**

▶ Chvostek's sign is associated with hypocalcemia and hypoparathyroidism. **(M-S)**

▶ A client who's receiving lithium should maintain adequate intake of salt and fluids. **(PSY)**

▶ The client with acute-angle glaucoma may complain of seeing a halo around lights or visual images. **(M-S)**

▶ Yellowing of vision is a symptom of digoxin toxicity. **(M-S)**

▶ To help a client compensate for the loss of peripheral vision, the nurse should instruct him to turn his head slowly to increase the visual field. **(M-S)**

▶ During an enema, the client may experience cramps if water flows into the colon too rapidly. If so, then slow the instillation rate. **(M-S)**

▶ A client with severe carbon monoxide poisoning may have cherry-red or pale, cyanotic skin. **(M-S)**

▶ With a physician's order, Credé's maneuver is used to help empty the bladder of a client with urinary retention. **(M-S)**

▶ A client with a history of basal cell carcinoma should avoid prolonged exposure to the sun. (M-S)

▶ During a bath, the nurse should prevent the client from becoming chilled. (FND)

▶ The neonate's transitional feces are loose and green to yellow. (MAT)

▶ By the fourth day after birth, the breast-fed neonate usually passes three to four light yellow feces daily. (MAT)

▶ During phototherapy, the neonate's feces are bright green as a result of increased excretion of bilirubin. (MAT)

▶ A client who has a C5 spinal injury can lift his shoulder and elbow to a limited degree but has no sensation below the clavicle. (M-S)

▶ When cleaning a wound, the nurse should wipe in only one direction, using a new gauze pad for each stroke. Don't wipe from edge to edge because doing so will bring contaminants into the wound. (M-S)

▶ Digoxin causes a slower, stronger heartbeat and allows the heart to rest between beats. (M-S)

▶ "Tet spells" are common in children with tetralogy of Fallot. (PED)

▶ Neonates usually undergo phenylketonuria testing 72 hours after birth, after consuming a protein feeding. (MAT)

▶ Stomach acid turns litmus paper to pink or red. (M-S)

▶ The nurse should use nitrazine paper to determine whether fluid that leaks from a pregnant woman's vagina is amniotic fluid. (MAT)

▶ The Tensilon (edrophonium) test is used to diagnose myasthenia gravis. (M-S)

▶ In a child with strabismus, the nondiverging eye should be patched. (PED)

▶ Colchicine is the drug of choice to treat acute gout. (M-S)

▶ To perform quadriceps sitting exercises, the client tries to push the popliteal space into the bed while raising his heel. (M-S)

▶ A *xenograft* is a skin graft that's made of tissue obtained from another species. (M-S)

▶ Sputum smear and culture provides a definitive diagnosis of tuberculosis. (M-S)

▶ A person who has a positive result on a test for human immunodeficiency virus (HIV) shouldn't keep a cat because of the risk of being exposed to toxoplasmosis. (M-S)

▶ Fat embolism usually occurs about 48 hours after a fracture and usually lodges in the lungs. **(M-S)**

▶ Complete protein foods, such as meat, dairy, fish, poultry, and eggs, contain adequate amounts of the nine essential amino acids. **(M-S)**

▶ In cheilosis, which is associated with riboflavin deficiency, cracks appear at the corners of the mouth. **(M-S)**

▶ A bland diet includes foods such as milk, cream, cereals, soup, rice, lean meats, fish, custards, and plain cake. **(M-S)**

▶ A medium-size apple provides 3.5 g of dietary fiber. **(FND)**

▶ Neonates of mothers who smoke are more likely to be small for gestational age than those of nonsmoking mothers. **(MAT)**

▶ When caring for a client who has chest tubes attached to suction, the nurse should keep a clamp at the bedside in case of emergency. **(M-S)**

▶ *Viability* is the ability of a fetus to live outside the womb. **(MAT)**

▶ In a high-risk pregnancy, certain conditions of the mother, such as advanced age or systemic disease, place the fetus or mother at increased risk for harm or adverse outcome. **(MAT)**

▶ Quickening is a presumptive sign of pregnancy. **(MAT)**

▶ Braxton Hicks contractions are a probable sign of pregnancy. **(MAT)**

▶ Signs of preeclampsia include edema, proteinuria, and increased blood pressure. **(MAT)**

▶ Magnesium sulfate is the drug of choice for clients who have gestational hypertension. **(MAT)**

▶ A bounding pulse indicates excess fluid volume. **(M-S)**

▶ If the client has frostbite, the nurse should rewarm the affected part gradually rather than massage the frozen extremities, fingers, or toes. **(M-S)**

▶ The nurse should teach the client who has a colostomy to lift the stoma appliance away from the stoma gently to permit gas to escape. **(M-S)**

▶ Cretinism is a congenital form of hypothyroidism. **(M-S)**

▶ In the client who has a C1 or C2 injury, respirations are maintained with a phrenic pacemaker. **(M-S)**

▶ *Gynecomastia* is overdeveloped breast tissue in a male. **(M-S)**

▶ Muscle weakness and cardiac arrhythmia are common in clients with hypokalemia or hyperkalemia. **(M-S)**

▶ A *bruit,* or rushing sound, heard with a stethoscope over the thyroid gland indicates a hypermetabolic state. **(FND)**

▶ Lower GI pain is usually a late symptom of colon cancer.   **(M-S)**

▶ To conserve energy in a client who's in a weakened state, the nurse may need to alternate care procedures with rest periods.   **(M-S)**

▶ Blood samples drawn before breakfast are usually more chemically uniform than those drawn later in the day.   **(M-S)**

▶ The nurse should use a 21G to 23G needle to withdraw blood.   **(FND)**

▶ When cleaning a puncture site before a needle aspiration, the nurse should clean from the center outward, using a circular motion.   **(FND)**

▶ After a bone marrow aspiration, slides of the material obtained must be sent uncontaminated to the laboratory immediately.   **(FND)**

▶ The drugs commonly used to treat myasthenia gravis include anticholinesterase medications such as pyridostigmine (Mestinon).   **(M-S)**

▶ Before bronchoscopy, the nurse should check the client for dentures and remove them.   **(M-S)**

▶ After bronchoscopy, the nurse should withhold foods and fluids until the client's gag reflex returns.   **(M-S)**

▶ After esophageal endoscopy, pain, difficulty swallowing, and fever may indicate perforation.   **(M-S)**

▶ Obesity is associated with increased insulin resistance.   **(M-S)**

▶ Oral antidiabetic agents stimulate the production of insulin.   **(M-S)**

▶ When taken orally, insulin is destroyed by gastric juices.   **(M-S)**

▶ Exercise lowers the blood glucose level by increasing insulin uptake by muscles and improving insulin use.   **(M-S)**

▶ In a client who's taking antipsychotic medications, constant motor activity is a classic sign of akathisia. (Think "A" for akathisia and "ants in the pants.")   **(PSY)**

▶ A *neologism* is a meaningless word or term coined by a person with psychosis.   **(PSY)**

▶ To administer gavage feedings to an infant, the nurse should use a gravity drip.   **(PED)**

▶ An oral airway should be kept at the bedside of a client who's on seizure precautions.   **(M-S)**

▶ Enterobiasis (pinworms) is most commonly diagnosed in a client who has anal itching.   **(M-S)**

▶ A low-fat diet is appropriate for a client with cholecystitis.   **(M-S)**

▶ A decreased vitamin K level causes a prolonged prothrombin time.   **(M-S)**

▶ Hydroxyzine pamoate (Vistaril) is given preoperatively to reduce the client's opioid requirements and to reduce anxiety. **(M-S)**

▶ A client who's taking metronidazole (Flagyl) may experience a metallic taste in his mouth and dark red-brown urine. **(M-S)**

▶ For the client with anorexia nervosa, correcting electrolyte imbalances is the most important nursing goal. **(PSY)**

▶ To prevent self-induced vomiting, the nurse should monitor the client with anorexia nervosa for 45 to 90 minutes after meals. **(PSY)**

▶ A dry delivery occurs when the fetus isn't delivered within 24 hours after rupture of the amniotic membranes. Mother and child are at risk for infection. **(MAT)**

▶ If the physician orders 5 lb (2.3 kg) of traction weight for a child in Bryant's traction, the nurse should place 2½-lb (1.1-kg) weights on each leg. **(PED)**

▶ For a child in Bryant's traction, a vest jacket or an abdominal restraint is used instead of elbow restraints. **(PED)**

▶ A mobile provides visual stimulation only and should be removed from the infant's bed when he reaches age 4 months. **(PED)**

▶ For a 5-year-old child who's confined to bed, effective diversional activities include playing with clay and drawing. **(PED)**

▶ A client who's taking disulfiram (Antabuse) should avoid alcohol and alcohol-containing products. **(M-S)**

▶ Disulfiram serves as aversion therapy for clients who intend to abstain from alcohol. **(PSY)**

▶ The nurse should administer lithium with meals to minimize GI upset. **(PSY)**

▶ Methylene blue (Urolene Blue) can turn urine and sometimes feces blue-green. **(M-S)**

▶ If a client's hair is matted with blood, the nurse should clean it with hydrogen peroxide to dissolve the blood and then rinse it with saline solution. **(M-S)**

▶ Before and after administering an opioid, the nurse must assess the client for respiratory depression. **(M-S)**

▶ The nurse should irrigate the client's eye from the inner to the outer canthus. **(M-S)**

▶ Before applying an eye ointment, the nurse should express a small amount of ointment onto a sterile gauze pad. **(M-S)**

▶ A bed cradle is used to keep bed sheets and blankets off of the client's feet to prevent footdrop or external rotation. **(M-S)**

▶ The three domains of learning are psychomotor, cognitive, and affective.
(FND)

▶ The neonatal period encompasses the first 28 days after birth.   (PED)

▶ *Fixation* is arrested development of the personality at a particular stage because of anxiety.   (PSY)

▶ At birth, the neonate's hearing is indistinct because of fluid retention in the middle ear.   (MAT)

▶ *Meconium* is the first fecal material passed by the neonate.   (MAT)

▶ For a neonate, normal urine output is 15 to 60 ml (½ to 2 oz) daily.   (MAT)

▶ Children younger than age 6 who have a history of pica are at risk for lead poisoning.   (PED)

▶ The four types of play are onlooker play, solitary play, parallel play, and associative play.   (PED)

▶ *Stereognosis* is the ability to identify an object by touch, as when a client with eyes closed can identify a coin placed in his hand as a quarter.   (FND)

▶ *Regression* is a return to an earlier stage of development.   (PED)

▶ Ovulation typically occurs 1 to 2 years after menarche.   (M-S)

▶ To prevent anemia, girls and women ages 10 to 55 should consume 18 mg of iron daily.   (M-S)

▶ *Menopause* is the cessation of menses.   (M-S)

▶ *Climacteric* is the cessation of reproductive functioning in women (menopause).   (M-S)

▶ Hot flashes may take the form of sweating, a sensation of heat in the chest, or sleep disturbances.   (M-S)

▶ Lentigo senilis, sometimes called "age spots" or "liver spots," result from clustering of melanocytes.   (M-S)

▶ According to the continuity theory, individuals maintain their values, morals, behavior, and habits as they age.   (FND)

▶ For optimal effectiveness, the nurse should administer antacids 1 hour after meals.   (M-S)

▶ Bone marrow suppression is a life-threatening risk associated with phenytoin (Dilantin) therapy.   (M-S)

▶ A client who takes insulin should avoid alcohol and aspirin unless these substances are approved by his physician.   (M-S)

▶ The nurse should warn the client who's receiving antipsychotic drug therapy to avoid activities that require alertness or good psychomotor control and to apply sunscreen before engaging in outdoor daylight activities.   **(PSY)**

▶ Withdrawal symptoms may occur in a client who abruptly stops taking barbiturates after long-term use.   **(M-S)**

▶ To relieve dry mouth, the nurse should provide sugarless hard candy, a mouth rinse, ice chips, or glycerin swabs (unless contraindicated).   **(M-S)**

▶ The client with a serum potassium level of less than 3 mEq/L needs potassium replacement therapy.   **(M-S)**

▶ To maintain constant hormone levels, thyroid hormone medication should be taken at the same time each day.   **(M-S)**

▶ Thyroid hormone medication should be stored in tight, light-resistant bottles.   **(M-S)**

▶ In Fowler's position, the head of the client's bed is elevated 45 to 90 degrees.   **(FND)**

▶ In the semi-Fowler or low Fowler position, the head of the bed is elevated 15 to 45 degrees.   **(FND)**

▶ In high Fowler's position, the head of the bed is elevated 90 degrees.   **(FND)**

▶ A client who's on nothing-by-mouth status can't receive ice chips to relieve dry mouth.   **(FND)**

▶ A vasectomy doesn't affect a man's sexual potency, erections, or semen ejaculation.   **(M-S)**

▶ The nurse who makes statements such as, "Don't worry," "You look better and better every day," or "You'll be fine" is providing false reassurance to the client, which blocks communication.   **(FND)**

▶ The nurse should follow the ABCDE rule to prioritize nursing actions: airway, breathing, circulation, disease process, and everything else.   **(FND)**

▶ A *retrospective audit* is an evaluation of nursing care after it has been delivered.   **(FND)**

▶ A *concurrent audit* is an evaluation of nursing care as it is being delivered.   **(FND)**

▶ In a *peer review,* a nurse evaluates the work performed by a nurse of equal status.   **(FND)**

▶ *Desquamation* is peeling of the skin.   **(M-S)**

▶ When caring for a client who's at risk for alcohol withdrawal, the nurse should monitor vital signs based on the client's status.   **(PSY)**

▶ Alcohol detoxification is most effective when it takes place in a structured environment with a supportive, nonjudgmental staff. **(PSY)**

▶ When caring for a client who's experiencing alcohol withdrawal, the nurse should maintain a calm environment, minimize intrusions, and eliminate shadows. **(PSY)**

▶ An alcoholic client requires folic acid, oral thiamine, multivitamins, and adequate food and fluid intake. **(PSY)**

▶ A client who's dependent on opiates typically has withdrawal symptoms within 12 hours after the last opiate dose. **(PSY)**

▶ A client with Crohn's disease should consume a bland, low-residue diet that's high in proteins, calories, and vitamins. **(M-S)**

▶ Chronic carriers of hepatitis B have positive results on tests for hepatitis B surface antigen, but have no signs of the disease. **(M-S)**

▶ Neurogenic bladder dysfunction results from conditions that affect bladder innervation. **(M-S)**

▶ Oxygen and carbon dioxide passively diffuse between alveoli and blood capillaries in the lungs. **(M-S)**

▶ When collecting 24-hour fractional urine specimens, the nurse should determine the number of bottles needed based on the collection period. **(M-S)**

▶ A Logan bar is used postoperatively in a child who's recovering from cleft-lip repair. **(PED)**

▶ Aortic stenosis causes a loud, rough systolic murmur over the aortic area. **(M-S)**

▶ *Elective surgery* is surgery that must be performed in the near future. **(M-S)**

▶ *Urgent surgery* is surgery that must be performed within 24 to 48 hours to prevent further harm. **(M-S)**

▶ *Emergency surgery* is surgery that must be performed immediately to save the client's life. **(M-S)**

▶ *Ambulatory surgery*, often called "outpatient" or "in-and-out" surgery, requires no overnight stay in the hospital. **(M-S)**

▶ Urine has an acidic pH, normally around 6.0. **(M-S)**

▶ About 85% of arterial emboli originate from thrombi in the heart chambers. **(M-S)**

▶ When caring for a client with an embolus in an arm or a leg, the nurse should keep the affected part at or below the horizontal plane of the body. **(M-S)**

▶ Drug administration is a dependent function of the nurse. **(FND)**

▶ Jaundice that arises during the first 24 hours after delivery signals erythroblastosis fetalis (pathologic jaundice).   **(MAT)**

▶ The nurse should instruct the outpatient to measure and record his pulse before taking verapamil.   **(M-S)**

▶ The client's urine is considered radioactive for 24 hours after radioisotope injection.   **(M-S)**

▶ The nurse should teach the client to take the oral antidiabetic drug chlorpropamide (Diabinese) in the morning.   **(M-S)**

▶ Salivary amylase triggers the digestion of starch.   **(M-S)**

▶ A client who has pain as a result of appendicitis should be placed in Fowler's position.   **(M-S)**

▶ Analgesics can mask the pain of a ruptured appendix.   **(M-S)**

▶ *Nursing malpractice* is negligence by a nurse that causes injury or harm to a client.   **(FND)**

▶ In true labor, the client typically has pain and discomfort first in the back and then in the abdomen.   **(MAT)**

▶ As a general rule, the nurse can't refuse a patient-care assignment.   **(FND)**

▶ To measure the height of a client who can't stand, the nurse should mark the bed sheet at the top of the client's head and at the bottom of the feet, and then measure the distance between the two marks.   **(FND)**

▶ In a client who has an esophageal balloon tamponade, back pain, upper abdominal pain, or shock suggests esophageal perforation.   **(M-S)**

▶ After reconstitution, a cephalosporin solution may change color if it's not used within 24 hours.   **(M-S)**

▶ Chloramphenicol antagonizes the bactericidal action of penicillin.   **(M-S)**

▶ A peripheral I.V. site should be changed every 48 to 72 hours.   **(M-S)**

▶ During the early stage of shock, the client's blood pressure may be normal, but respiratory and heart rates increase. As shock continues, the heart and lungs can't compensate, and blood pressure begins to fall.   **(M-S)**

▶ Cool, moist, pale skin, as seen during shock, results from diversion of blood from the skin to major organs.   **(M-S)**

▶ To assess capillary refill, the nurse applies pressure over the nail bed until blanching occurs, quickly releases the pressure, and notes how quickly blanching fades (less than 3 seconds is normal).   **(M-S)**

▶ The nursing process is a systematic, problem-solving method of providing nursing care.   **(FND)**

▶ When giving an insulin injection, the nurse should use a 25G ⅝″ needle.
(M-S)

▶ Residual urine (urine that remains in the bladder after voiding) normally measures 50 to 100 ml. (M-S)

▶ Assessment starts with the nurse's first encounter with the client and continues throughout the health history interview and physical examination.
(FND)

▶ During the planning stage of the nursing process, the nurse formulates and prioritizes nursing diagnoses, defines goals and expected outcomes, and develops the care plan. (FND)

▶ During implementation, the nurse puts the care plan into action by carrying out specific nursing actions and evaluating the client's responses. (FND)

▶ During evaluation, the nurse determines whether the outcome criteria specified in the care plan have been met and, if needed, modifies the plan. (FND)

▶ Pulse oximetry measures oxygenated hemoglobin in the blood. (FND)

▶ Cottage cheese contains about 150 mg of calcium per cup, making it an excellent source of calcium. (FND)

▶ An acceptable level of cholesterol is less than 200 mg/dL in women and less than 190 mg/dL in men. (FND)

▶ In total incontinence, the client has an unpredictable loss of urine. In bowel incontinence, the client has an involuntary loss of feces. (FND)

▶ The tonsils and adenoids are the first line of defense against respiratory infection. (M-S)

▶ A spermatozoon contributes either an X or a Y chromosome. (MAT)

▶ In a client with glaucoma, a miotic such as pilocarpine is used three to four times daily to constrict the pupil and open Schlemm's canal. (M-S)

▶ Weight gain is the most reliable indicator of a positive response to total parenteral nutrition therapy. (M-S)

▶ The nurse should suspect thrombophlebitis in a client with Homans' sign.
(M-S)

▶ When preparing for urinary catheterization, the nurse should place a female client in the dorsal recumbent position with knees bent. (M-S)

▶ The two phases of metabolism are anabolism and catabolism. (M-S)

▶ *Anabolism* refers to metabolic reactions that are essential for growth and repair. (M-S)

▶ *Catabolism* refers to metabolic reactions that break down larger molecules to smaller ones to produce fuel for the body. (M-S)

▶ In elderly clients, the most common cause of hyperthyroidism is toxic nodular goiter.　**(M-S)**

▶ The body processes foods in the following sequence: ingestion, digestion, absorption, transport, cell metabolism, and excretion.　**(M-S)**

▶ Dietary fiber, or roughage, is derived from cellulose.　**(M-S)**

▶ The body metabolizes alcohol at a fixed rate.　**(M-S)**

▶ The alcohol concentration (proof) of a beverage indicates the percentage of alcohol multiplied by two.　**(M-S)**

▶ The liver metabolizes about 90% of ingested alcohol by using vitamin B to detoxify the alcohol (100-proof alcohol is 50% alcohol).　**(M-S)**

▶ Proteins make up the major portion of muscles, bones, skin, and hair.　**(M-S)**

▶ Skin-fold thickness reflects the amount of subcutaneous adipose tissue.　**(M-S)**

▶ Red blood cells transport hemoglobin.　**(FND)**

▶ White blood cells fight infection.　**(FND)**

▶ Platelets form a hemostatic plug.　**(FND)**

▶ *Hemophilia* is an X-linked recessive bleeding disorder that's passed from a mother to her son.　**(M-S)**

▶ *Von Willebrand's disease* is caused by platelet dysfunction and factor VIII deficiency. It's more common in females than in males and may resolve on its own as the child ages.　**(M-S)**

▶ *Sickle cell anemia* is a chronic hemolytic anemia that's caused by hemoglobin S, a defective hemoglobin.　**(M-S)**

▶ *Petechiae* are tiny, round, red or purplish spots that may appear on the skin and mucous membranes.　**(M-S)**

▶ *Purpura* is a general term that's used to describe a purplish skin discoloration caused by extravasation of blood.　**(M-S)**

▶ Lavender-top tubes contain edetate, an anticoagulant; they are used to collect a sample of whole blood.　**(M-S)**

▶ Red-top tubes contain no additives; they are used to collect serum samples.　**(M-S)**

▶ Blue-top tubes contain sodium citrate and citric acid; they are used to collect plasma for coagulation studies.　**(M-S)**

▶ Gray-top tubes contain glycolytic inhibitor; they are usually used to determine serum glucose.　**(M-S)**

▶ Black-top tubes contain sodium oxalate; they are used to collect blood for co-agulation studies.   (M-S)

▶ Green-top tubes contain heparin; they are used to collect serum samples for several studies.   (M-S)

▶ Heinz bodies in red blood cells indicate glucose-6-phosphate dehydrogenase deficiency.   (M-S)

▶ Clients usually receive a sedative 1 hour before a bone marrow biopsy. (M-S)

▶ A butterfly rash across the bridge of the nose is a classic sign of systemic lupus erythematosus (SLE).   (M-S)

▶ A blood sample used for serum lithium measurement should be drawn im-mediately before the client is to receive the next lithium dose, or 8 to 12 hours after the last dose.   (PSY)

▶ For a man, the normal daily caloric requirement is 2,300 to 3,100 calories.
                                                                        (M-S)

▶ For a woman, the normal daily caloric requirement is 1,600 to 2,400 calories.
                                                                        (M-S)

▶ *Desensitization therapy,* a process of slowly exposing the client to a feared stim-uli, is used to treat phobic disorders.   (PSY)

▶ During nasotracheal suctioning, the nurse should maintain the infant's head in a neutral position by placing the infant on his back, with a towel under his shoulders.   (PED)

▶ The nurse should suction an infant for no more than 5 to 10 seconds at a time, pausing for 1 to 3 minutes between each suctioning period.   (PED)

▶ The umbilical cord is tied off and cut about 1" (2.5 cm) from the abdominal wall unless the infant is born in an emergent situation outside the hospital. In that case, the cord is cut at 6" (15 cm).   (MAT)

▶ An *ectopic pregnancy* is an abnormal pregnancy in which the ovum implants out-side the uterus.   (MAT)

▶ The first stage of labor starts with the onset of contractions and ends with full dilation.   (MAT)

▶ The second stage of labor ends with delivery of the neonate.   (MAT)

▶ The third stage of labor ends with expulsion of the placenta.   (MAT)

▶ In a full-term neonate, the heel crease extends two-thirds of the way up the length of the heel; in a preterm neonate, the crease extends less than two-thirds of this distance.   (MAT)

▶ Throughout pregnancy, a woman's blood volume increases, but her blood pressure should remain constant or slightly lower than her baseline.   (MAT)

▶ *Hegar's sign* is a probable sign of pregnancy. (MAT)

▶ The *multiparous woman* is one who has given birth to two or more children. (MAT)

▶ The *primigravida* is a woman in her first pregnancy. (MAT)

▶ *Goodell's sign* is a softening of the cervix, a probable sign of pregnancy. (MAT)

▶ *Melasma,* or *chloasma,* is a tan or brownish pigmentation on the face, especially the cheeks and nose, that commonly occurs in pregnant women. (MAT)

▶ *Linea nigra* is a dark line from the mons pubis to the umbilicus that commonly appears during pregnancy because of an increase in the hormone melanotropin. (MAT)

▶ Presumptive signs of pregnancy are the least indicative signs, and could indicate other conditions. (MAT)

▶ Probable signs of pregnancy can be documented by the examiner. (MAT)

▶ Three fetal cardiac structures disappear after birth: the ductus venosus, foramen ovale, and ductus arteriosus. (MAT)

▶ The examiner can hear the fetal heartbeat with a Doppler device as early as the 10th to 12th week of pregnancy. (MAT)

▶ At 12 to 14 weeks' gestation, the uterine fundus is palpable over the symphysis pubis and is considered an abdominal organ. (MAT)

▶ At 36 weeks' gestation, the uterus is at the level of the xiphoid process. (MAT)

▶ For a pelvic examination, the nurse should place the client in the lithotomy position. (M-S)

▶ Rubella poses the greatest risk to the embryo or fetus in the first 2 to 8 weeks of pregnancy. (MAT)

▶ Live-virus vaccines are contraindicated during pregnancy. (MAT)

▶ Pregnant clients should avoid oral anticoagulants because these agents cross the placenta. Heparin sulfate is a Category C drug and may be used in pregnant women when its potential benefits outweigh its risks. (MAT)

▶ *Effleurage* is a relaxation technique that can help to distract the pregnant client and reduce her pain. (MAT)

▶ Spontaneous abortion and ectopic pregnancy are the most common causes of bleeding during the first trimester. (MAT)

▶ The force of labor is supplied by the uterine fundus and implemented by uterine contractions. (MAT)

▶ At 20 weeks' gestation, the uterine fundus should be at the level of the umbilicus. **(MAT)**

▶ At 40 weeks' gestation, the uterine fundus is typically about 1½" (4 cm) below the xiphoid process as a result of lightening. **(MAT)**

▶ A neonate whose gestational age is less than 38 weeks is considered premature. **(MAT)**

▶ *Linea alba* is a white line that runs from the mons pubis to the umbilicus in some pregnant women. **(MAT)**

▶ After a client has a tonsillectomy, the nurse should suction out viscous mucus and provide warm saline gargles every 1 to 2 hours to relieve pain, promote comfort, and help eliminate foul breath odor. **(M-S)**

▶ Immediately after surgery, the client should be placed in a side-lying position unless contraindicated and an emesis basin should be used to catch drainage and secretions until the client is fully alert. **(M-S)**

▶ Bright red, moderate vaginal bleeding without cramping or cervical dilation signals a threatened abortion. **(MAT)**

▶ *Complete abortion* occurs when all products of conception are expelled spontaneously without assistance. **(MAT)**

▶ *Hydramnios* is excessive amniotic fluid formation (more than 2,000 ml). **(MAT)**

▶ Excessive intake of vitamin K (from eating large amounts of leafy green vegetables) decreases the anticoagulant effect of warfarin (Coumadin). **(M-S)**

▶ After giving an injection, the nurse shouldn't recap the needle but should discard it in the appropriate container. **(FND)**

▶ According to Freud, the genital stage of psychosexual development occurs from ages 12 to 20. **(PED)**

▶ According to Erikson, the stage of identity versus role confusion takes place from ages 13 to 18. **(PED)**

▶ *Tolerance* is increasing resistance to the usual effects of a particular drug because of continued use. **(M-S)**

▶ The antidote for heparin overdose is protamine sulfate. **(M-S)**

▶ The antidote for warfarin (Coumadin) overdose is vitamin K. **(M-S)**

▶ A gallium scan may be used to detect primary or metastatic cancer. **(M-S)**

▶ On a child, mitt restraints should be removed at least twice each shift so that the child can exercise his fingers. **(PED)**

▶ Bell's palsy is caused by inflammation of cranial nerve VII (the facial nerve). **(M-S)**

▶ In a nonreactive nonstress test, the fetal heart rate doesn't increase with fetal movement, or fewer than five such responses occur in 20 minutes.   (MAT)

▶ In a reactive nonstress test, the fetal heart rate increases by 15 beats/minute above the baseline in response to fetal activity, with five such responses occurring in 20 minutes.   (MAT)

▶ The physician may order a nonstress test for a pregnant client who has a prolonged pregnancy (more than 41 weeks' gestation), diabetes, or a history of poor pregnancy outcomes or of intrauterine fetal death.   (MAT)

▶ When feeding an infant who has a tracheostomy tube, the nurse should cover the opening with a moist gauze pad or a bib to prevent food or fluid from falling into the opening.   (PED)

▶ When changing the ties on a tracheostomy tube, the nurse should leave the old ties in place until the new ones are applied.   (M-S)

▶ The nurse should obtain help from another nurse when changing the ties on an infant's tracheostomy tube.   (PED)

▶ If an intradermal tuberculin skin test dose is injected too deep, as evidenced by the absence of a wheal, the nurse should inject another dose at a site 2″ (5 cm) away.   (M-S)

▶ An intradermal tuberculin skin test should be read in 48 to 72 hours, when the induration is most evident.   (M-S)

▶ The normal specific gravity of urine is 1.010 to 1.025.   (M-S)

▶ When diagnosed early, cervical cancer has a cure rate of 95% or more. (M-S)

▶ Tuberculin skin tests are based on the principle of delayed hypersensitivity.   (M-S)

▶ An example of a hypotonic solution is 0.33% sodium chloride solution.   (M-S)

▶ Signs of hypernatremia include dry, sticky mucous membranes and a red, swollen tongue.   (M-S)

▶ A pureed diet is usually given to clients who have difficulty chewing or swallowing food.   (M-S)

▶ The oxygen concentration of room air is 21%.   (M-S)

▶ After a barium enema, the nurse should encourage the client to drink more fluids to enhance barium elimination.   (M-S)

▶ Proteinuria commonly indicates glomerular injury. If the urine contains albumin, expect edema in the body.   (M-S)

▶ A *delusion* is a fixed false belief that persists and can't be corrected by reason.   (PSY)

▶ An obstructed bile duct impairs the absorption of nutrients and fat-soluble vitamins. (M-S)

▶ When mixing regular insulin with intermediate- or long-acting insulin, the nurse should draw regular insulin into the syringe first (after injecting the correct amount of air into the intermediate- or long-acting insulin vial). (M-S)

▶ After completing the assessment and nursing diagnosis steps of the nursing process, the nurse formulates goals (outcomes). (FND)

▶ Assessing capillary refill is one way to check the circulatory status of a casted extremity. (M-S)

▶ When performing venipuncture, the nurse should select the most distal vein in the client's hand, arm, leg, or foot. (M-S)

▶ All clients older than age 65 should be assessed for aneurysm because of the normal vascular changes that accompany aging. (M-S)

▶ Tinnitus is a sign of salicylate (aspirin) toxicity. (M-S)

▶ Ulcers associated with Buerger's disease heal slowly. (M-S)

▶ Raynaud's disease is characterized by recurrent inflammation of the intermediate small veins of the extremities. (M-S)

▶ As Raynaud's disease progresses, the client may have ulcers and superficial gangrene of the hands. (M-S)

▶ *OU* denotes each eye or both eyes, *OD* denotes the right eye, and *OS* denotes the left eye. (FND)

▶ Applesauce thickens stools. (PED)

▶ When removing a foreign body from the client's eye, the nurse should irrigate the eye with sterile normal saline solution. (M-S)

▶ For the client with a corneal injury caused by a caustic substance, emergency care involves copious flushing of the eye with water. (M-S)

▶ To remove an artificial eye, the nurse should pull down on the client's lower lid and exert slight pressure on the eyelid to overcome the suction that holds the eye in place. (FND)

▶ The nurse should use normal saline solution to clean an artificial eye. (FND)

▶ Cataract surgery removes the lens of the client's eye. (M-S)

▶ Severe pain after cataract surgery indicates increased intraocular pressure. (M-S)

▶ After performing irrigation of the ear, the nurse should place the client on the affected side to allow remaining fluid to drain. (M-S)

▶ *Ascites* is excess fluid in the peritoneal cavity. (M-S)

► A *thready pulse* is a pulse that's fine and barely perceptible. **(FND)**

► If the client with an indwelling urinary catheter has abdominal discomfort, the nurse should check for bladder distention. **(M-S)**

► An indwelling urinary catheter that's improperly positioned and secured may cause bladder or urethral injury. **(M-S)**

► The nurse who accidentally inserts a urinary catheter into the client's vagina should leave the catheter in place temporarily while starting the procedure again with a new catheter. **(M-S)**

► When assessing a client with burns, the nurse should use the Rule of Nines to estimate the extent of burn and the percentage of body surface area burned. **(M-S)**

► A *partial-thickness burn* involves the epidermis and part of the dermis. **(M-S)**

► Taking the axillary temperature is the least accurate way to measure body temperature. **(FND)**

► After suctioning, the nurse must document the color, amount, consistency, and odor of secretions as well as the client's tolerance for the procedure. **(M-S)**

► The abbreviation for "after meals" is *p.c.* **(FND)**

► After a bladder irrigation, the nurse should document the amount, color, clarity, and appearance of clots or sediment in the urine. **(M-S)**

► Placement in the semi-Fowler position, diaphragmatic breathing, and relaxation are essential treatment measures in a client who's experiencing an asthma attack. **(M-S)**

► Prostate cancer commonly metastasizes to the bone, lymph nodes, brain, and lungs. **(M-S)**

► A needle's gauge indicates its diameter; the larger the gauge, the smaller the diameter. **(FND)**

► After turning a client, the nurse should document the position to which the client was turned, the time at which turning occurred, and the findings of skin assessment. **(M-S)**

► In a client with increasing intracranial pressure, the level of consciousness is the most significant indicator of health status. **(M-S)**

► The acronym *PERRLA* means pupils equal, round, react to light, and accommodation. **(FND)**

► When percussing the client's chest during postural drainage, the nurse should cup her hands and percuss for $1\frac{1}{2}$ to 2 minutes over each lobe. **(M-S)**

► Regular insulin is the only type of insulin that can be mixed with other insulins. **(M-S)**

► When taking a client's radial pulse, the nurse should assess its rate, rhythm, quality, and force. **(FND)**

► When documenting respirations, the nurse should include their rate, rhythm, depth, and quality. **(FND)**

► For a subcutaneous injection, the nurse should use a 25G ⁵/₈" needle. **(FND)**

► The nurse should use passive range-of-motion exercises for the unconscious client. **(M-S)**

► The nurse's notation *AA + O × 3* means that the client is awake and alert and oriented to person, place, and time. **(FND)**

► The respiratory center is located in the medulla oblongata. **(M-S)**

► Usually, foods and fluids are withheld for 8 hours before excretory urography. **(M-S)**

► After administering an intradermal injection, the nurse shouldn't massage the injection site. **(FND)**

► When administering an intradermal injection, the nurse should hold the syringe almost parallel to the client's skin, with the needle bevel up. **(FND)**

► After thyroidectomy, the client should be placed in the semi-Fowler position, with the head firmly supported by pillows (usually cervical pillows). **(M-S)**

► To obtain an accurate blood pressure reading, the nurse should pump the bulb until the mercury column or aneroid dial reaches 20 to 30 mm Hg before the point at which the pulse disappears or above the client's baseline systolic pressure. **(FND)**

► Before giving castor oil to prepare a client for a barium enema, the nurse may offer ice chips to minimize the unpleasant taste. **(M-S)**

► If a stoma is much lighter in color than it was when last assessed, the nurse should suspect decreased circulation to the stoma. **(M-S)**

► A client who has histrionic personality disorder displays manipulative behavior and dramatic emotional responses. **(PSY)**

► The nurse shouldn't massage a leg with a blood clot because doing so may dislodge the clot. **(M-S)**

► Jaundice is usually first detected by assessing the sclerae. **(M-S)**

► Jaundice is caused by a high serum bilirubin level. **(M-S)**

► Mydriatic drugs dilate the pupils. (Think "D" for mydriatic and dilate.) **(M-S)**

► Miotic drugs constrict the pupils. **(M-S)**

▶ After eye surgery, the nurse should place the client on the unaffected side. (M-S)

▶ Infectious mononucleosis is called the "kissing disease" because it's transmitted by oral secretions. (M-S)

▶ A client who's recovering from mononucleosis should stay in bed during periods of fever and should get additional rest at regular intervals. (M-S)

▶ Until recovery is complete, a client who has mononucleosis should avoid strenuous activity and competitive sports. The enlarged spleen is vulnerable to injury and may rupture as a result of even mild trauma. (M-S)

▶ Skin traction applies direct pulling force to the skeleton and is most effective in children who have healthy skin tissue. (M-S)

▶ When placing a nitroglycerin patch on a client, the nurse should avoid touching the medicated disk and should wash her hands after application; however, gloves aren't required. (M-S)

▶ When caring for a client with burns, the nurse should wear gloves, gown, mask, and protective headgear. (M-S)

▶ Before performing care procedures on a client with burns, the nurse should administer prescribed pain medication. (M-S)

▶ The nurse should count an irregular pulse for 1 full minute. (FND)

▶ A client who has a gastric ulcer should avoid aspirin and aspirin-containing products because they irritate the gastric mucosa. (M-S)

▶ If a client starts to vomit while lying in a supine position, the nurse should place the client on his side immediately and maintain a patent airway. (M-S)

▶ A sitz bath usually lasts about 20 minutes. (M-S)

▶ The Apgar score is used to assess the neonate's vital functions; it is obtained at 1 minute and at 5 minutes after delivery. (MAT)

▶ After feeding an infant who has had surgery to repair a cleft lip or palate, the nurse should rinse the infant's mouth with sterile water. (PED)

▶ An infant who has undergone surgery to repair a cleft palate is at increased risk for otitis media. (PED)

▶ Surgical repair of a cleft palate is usually performed when the infant is age 4 to 6 months and always before defective speech patterns develop. (PED)

▶ A cleft lip can be surgically corrected shortly after birth, but surgery may be delayed until the infant is age 1 to 3 months. (PED)

▶ When administering oral medication to an infant who has undergone surgery to correct a cleft lip or palate, the nurse should place the medication to one side of the mouth. (PED)

▶ Imaginative play is common in children around age 4. **(PED)**

▶ *Negativism* (saying "no" when "yes" would be a better response) is characteristic of toddlers. **(PED)**

▶ A child with ascites caused by chronic liver disease should be placed in the semi-Fowler position. **(PED)**

▶ Autistic children don't show normal attachment behaviors. **(PED)**

▶ Toilet training is usually successful during toddlerhood. **(PED)**

▶ Applying erythromycin ointment to the neonate's eyes helps prevent gonorrheal conjunctivitis. **(MAT)**

▶ Gonorrhea rarely causes symptoms in women or girls. **(M-S)**

▶ According to Erikson, the preschooler's developmental task is to gain initiative without experiencing guilt. **(PED)**

▶ Erythromycin ointment, which is used to prevent gonorrheal conjunctivitis in neonates, also eliminates chlamydia. **(M-S)**

▶ During the initial interview of a client diagnosed with syphilis, the nurse should identify the client's sexual contacts. Treatment should not be withheld if he refuses to identify them. **(M-S)**

▶ When suctioning the oral cavity and nasopharynx, the nurse should use a #5 to #8 French catheter in infants and a #8 to #10 French catheter in children. **(PED)**

▶ For nasotracheal suctioning, the nurse should set the suction regulator at 60 to 80 mm Hg for infants and at 95 to 115 mm Hg for children. **(PED)**

▶ The home-care nurse should remove all smoking material, such as matches, cigarettes, or cigars, from the room of a client who's receiving home oxygen therapy. She should also place a "no smoking" sign prominently in the room. **(M-S)**

▶ Flavoxate (Urispas) is used mainly as a urinary tract antispasmodic. **(M-S)**

▶ The signs and symptoms of cardiogenic shock result from loss of myocardial contractility, which in turn reduces cardiac output. **(M-S)**

▶ Hypovolemic shock leads to increased pulse rate, decreased systolic blood pressure, cold and clammy skin, pallor, thirst, altered mental status, and decreased urine output. **(M-S)**

▶ Life-threatening arrhythmias are common during the first 24 hours after a myocardial infarction. **(M-S)**

▶ For the client who has had a myocardial infarction, meticulous monitoring of fluid balance is crucial. **(M-S)**

▶ Cardiac output is determined by multiplying the stroke volume by the heart rate for 1 minute. **(M-S)**

▶ After a myocardial infarction, creatine kinase is the first enzyme level to increase. **(M-S)**

▶ The nurse should use normal saline solution to irrigate a nasogastric (NG) tube. **(M-S)**

▶ If a client who has an NG tube complains of a sore nostril, the nurse should apply a water-soluble lubricant. **(M-S)**

▶ The nurse may give the client anesthetic lozenges or use gargles to relieve a sore throat that's caused by irritation from an NG tube. **(M-S)**

▶ During the first 12 to 24 hours after gastric surgery, suctioned stomach contents appear brown from bleeding during surgery. **(M-S)**

▶ The lactate dehydrogenase level rises within 12 hours after the onset of a myocardial infarction. **(M-S)**

▶ After a myocardial infarction, cardiac enzyme levels rise; the higher they rise and the longer they remain at peak levels, the more serious the damage to heart muscle. **(M-S)**

▶ The nurse should use low intermittent suction when suctioning an NG tube. **(M-S)**

▶ When documenting drainage on a surgical dressing, the nurse should note its amount, color, and consistency. **(M-S)**

▶ In rare cases, electroconvulsive therapy (ECT) causes arrhythmias and even death. **(PSY)**

▶ Confusion and memory loss (called postshock amnesia) are among the most common mental status changes that occur after ECT. **(PSY)**

▶ Classic signs of pyloric stenosis are a palpable, olive-sized mass in the right upper abdominal quadrant, visible strong peristalsis that moves from left to right after feeding, and projectile vomiting. **(PED)**

▶ Valvular venous insufficiency is the most likely cause of varicose veins. **(M-S)**

▶ A client who has a colostomy should restrict his intake of fatty and fibrous foods and avoid foods that can obstruct the stoma. **(M-S)**

▶ During chemotherapy, a client who has a depressed white blood cell count should follow neutropenic precautions. **(M-S)**

▶ A client who has mitral valve stenosis typically has signs and symptoms associated with improper emptying of the left atrium and subsequent pulmonary congestion. **(M-S)**

▶ Mitral valve stenosis usually arises as a complication of rheumatic fever.
(M-S)

▶ If a chest tube becomes disconnected, the nurse should clamp the tube immediately with a Kelly clamp. (M-S)

▶ *Atelectasis* is an abnormal condition that's characterized by the collapse of lung tissue and incomplete expansion of lobules (clusters of alveoli) or a lung segment. (M-S)

▶ To perform cardiopulmonary resuscitation, the nurse should place the victim on a flat, solid surface. (M-S)

▶ Antacids interfere with the absorption of histamine-receptor antagonists.
(M-S)

▶ A client who has an ileal conduit should be instructed to empty the collection device before it's half full to prevent accidental, unplanned emptying. (M-S)

▶ To assess a client for a distended bladder, the nurse should check for a rounded mass above the pubis. (M-S)

▶ To test for Babinski's reflex, the nurse firmly strokes the lateral aspect of the client's sole. A positive response occurs when the client dorsiflexes the big toe and extends and fans the other toes. (M-S)

▶ A positive human immunodeficiency virus test result indicates that the client has been infected with the virus that causes acquired immunodeficiency syndrome (AIDS) and not that the client has AIDS. (M-S)

▶ Because human immunodeficiency virus appears in breast milk, it can be transmitted by breast-feeding. (MAT)

▶ For a client with heart failure, decreasing the workload of the heart (as by placing the client on bed rest) is one of the nurse's most important goals. (M-S)

▶ Performing meticulous skin care and turning the bedridden client every 2 hours are the most effective ways to prevent skin breakdown. (M-S)

▶ The nurse should suspect an asthma attack in a client who wheezes, coughs, or exhibits respiratory distress. (M-S)

▶ The nurse should advise a client who has an ileostomy to eat foods that deodorize the GI tract, such as spinach and parsley. (M-S)

▶ After adrenalectomy, decreased steroid production may lead to extensive loss of sodium and water. (M-S)

▶ During the first 24 hours after delivery, many women have a low-grade fever as a result of dehydration caused by labor. (MAT)

▶ Antiembolism stockings provide gradual compression of the superficial blood vessels, helping to prevent thrombus formation. (M-S)

▶ A client who no longer requires bed rest after a femoral-popliteal bypass graft should be permitted to walk and stand.   (M-S)

▶ The nurse should record ice chips as fluid intake at about one-half their volume (120 ml of ice chips should be recorded as 50 ml of water).   (M-S)

▶ Of the five senses, hearing is believed to be the last sense lost by comatose clients.   (M-S)

▶ In an adult, the most convenient veins for venipuncture are the basilic and median cubital veins.   (M-S)

▶ The drug zidovudine (AZT) is used to prevent replication of human immuno-deficiency virus.   (M-S)

▶ *Pneumocystis carinii* pneumonia is an opportunistic infection that's associated with acquired immunodeficiency syndrome.   (M-S)

▶ If a radioactive implant becomes dislodged, the nurse should retrieve the implant with tongs and place it in a lead-shielded container.   (M-S)

▶ A client who's receiving external radiation therapy should pat the irradiated skin dry.   (M-S)

▶ The nurse should give aluminum hydroxide separately and at least 1 hour before or after the administration of enteric-coated medications.   (M-S)

▶ By age 12 months, an infant has typically tripled his birth weight and has eight teeth.   (PED)

▶ If the umbilical cord is delivered before the fetus, don't attempt to place it back in the vagina. Instead, positively ventilate the fetus.   (MAT)

▶ *Buffers* are substances in the blood that prevent body fluid from becoming overly acidic or alkaline.   (M-S)

▶ Metabolic acidosis results from excessive loss of bicarbonate or excessive production or retention of acid.   (M-S)

▶ In *homonymous hemianopsia*, blindness occurs in the same half (right or left) of both the client's visual fields. Place all client items within this field of vision.   (M-S)

▶ After a total hip replacement, full weight bearing is restricted for 3 to 6 months.   (M-S)

▶ After a total knee replacement, the physician determines how soon the client is allowed to bear weight.   (M-S)

▶ Before giving an intermittent tube feeding, the nurse should verify that the tube is placed correctly.   (M-S)

▶ People who have type O blood are known as *universal donors*.   (FND)

▶ People who have type AB blood are known as *universal recipients*.   (FND)

▶ Nausea, vomiting, restlessness, and twitching are signs of disequilibrium syndrome caused by a rapid fluid shift. (M-S)

▶ In "setting sun," a sign of increased intracranial pressure, the iris is displaced downward and the sclera appears above the iris. (PED)

▶ The most effective use of electroconvulsive therapy is the treatment of clients who have severe depression. (PSY)

▶ For electroconvulsive therapy to be effective, the client should receive a total of 6 to 12 treatments. Usually, two or three treatments are given per week. (PSY)

▶ Return of reflex activity in the extremities below the level of injury indicates that spinal shock is resolving. (M-S)

▶ When caring for a client who has stomatitis, the nurse should provide frequent mouth care. (M-S)

▶ Hearing protection is required when sound intensity increases to more than 84 decibels. (M-S)

▶ In *otitis media*, the client typically has a bright red tympanic membrane and an absent light reflex (cone of light). (M-S)

▶ In *pericardiocentesis*, blood is withdrawn from the pericardial sac. (M-S)

▶ During labor, the resting phase between each contraction should last at least 30 seconds. (MAT)

▶ Urticaria is one of the first signs of a hemolytic transfusion reaction. (M-S)

▶ During peritoneal dialysis, return of brown dialysate indicates bowel perforation. (M-S)

▶ Early signs and symptoms of ketoacidosis include polyuria, polyphagia, fatigue, malaise, drowsiness, headache, and abdominal pain. (M-S)

▶ In an infant who has hydrocephalus, a shrill, high-pitched cry signals increasing intracranial pressure. (PED)

▶ *Prothrombin* is a clotting factor that's produced by the liver. (M-S)

▶ If a client is menstruating when a urine sample is collected, the nurse should make a note on the laboratory request. (M-S)

▶ During a lumbar puncture, the client should refrain from holding his breath to prevent interfering with pressure readings. (M-S)

▶ The rash associated with scarlet fever starts 12 to 48 hours after the onset of pharyngeal symptoms. (M-S)

▶ The recommended adult dose of sucralfate (Carafate) is 1 g (1 tablet) four times daily, taken on an empty stomach. (M-S)

▶ *Lochia rubra* is the vaginal discharge that occurs during the first 3 days post-partum. **(MAT)**

▶ *Lochia serosa* is the serous pink or brown vaginal discharge that appears from days 3 to 7 postpartum. **(MAT)**

▶ *Lochia alba* is the white discharge that occurs from days 7 to 10 postpartum and may last as long as 6 weeks. **(MAT)**

▶ The client should have nothing by mouth after midnight on the day before any surgery that involves general anesthesia. **(M-S)**

▶ A client who has inhaled smoke should be hospitalized for 24 hours to allow observation for delayed development of tracheal edema. **(M-S)**

▶ After a burn, two stages of physiologic changes occur: the hypovolemic stage and the diuretic stage. **(M-S)**

▶ When administering total parenteral nutrition by peripheral line, the nurse should change the tubing at least every 24 hours and should change the needle and dressing over the insertion site every 72 hours. **(M-S)**

▶ Colostrum is the thin, yellow fluid that's secreted by the breasts during pregnancy and the first postpartum days before lactation starts. **(MAT)**

▶ From a prepregnancy length of about $2\frac{1}{2}''$ (6.4 cm), the uterus grows to about $12\frac{1}{2}''$ (32 cm) at term. **(MAT)**

▶ The diagonal conjugate diameter of the pelvis is measured directly and used to estimate the true conjugate diameter. **(MAT)**

▶ Fetal heart tones are the most reliable indicator of fetal status. **(MAT)**

▶ The nurse should use standard precautions when caring for a client who has tuberculosis. **(M-S)**

▶ When performing pin care for a client who's in skeletal traction, the nurse's highest priority is to prevent osteomyelitis. **(M-S)**

▶ For the client with carbon monoxide poisoning, the nurse should administer humidified oxygen until the carboxyhemoglobin level is less than 5%. **(M-S)**

▶ The sweat chloride test is used to confirm a diagnosis of cystic fibrosis. **(PED)**

▶ The nurse should avoid giving routine I.M. injections into edematous tissue because the medication may not be absorbed. **(M-S)**

▶ In a client who's receiving dialysis, a palpated thrill or an auscultated bruit indicates that the internal shunt is working. **(M-S)**

▶ Early signs of acquired immunodeficiency syndrome (AIDS) include flulike symptoms, such as fatigue, night sweats, enlarged lymph nodes, anorexia, weight loss, pallor, and fever. **(M-S)**

▶ Late decelerations of the fetal heart rate indicate uteroplacental insufficiency.
                                                                            (MAT)

▶ During the manic phase of bipolar affective disorder, the nurse should protect the client from self-injury or exhaustion.   (PSY)

▶ To control the rapid emergence of the fetus's head during an emergency delivery, the nurse should place a hand on the head of the fetus and apply only enough pressure to guide the descent.   (MAT)

▶ Multiparous clients are at greater risk for postpartum bleeding than are primiparous clients.   (MAT)

▶ Safety of the client is the primary concern when planning care for a client with Alzheimer's disease.   (M-S)

▶ The client is usually the best source of health history information.   (FND)

▶ A client who has Parkinson's disease usually receives levodopa (Dopar) to compensate for dopamine deficiency.   (M-S)

▶ Clients who have multiple sclerosis are at increased risk for pressure ulcers.
                                                                            (M-S)

▶ Palliative therapy is used to relieve or reduce symptoms; it doesn't produce a cure.   (M-S)

▶ Pill-rolling tremors are a classic sign of Parkinson's disease.   (M-S)

▶ For the client who has Parkinson's disease, an important nursing goal is to improve mobility and help the client gain independence in self-care.   (M-S)

▶ Blood urea nitrogen normally measures 10 to 20 mg/dl.   (M-S)

▶ Metrorrhagia (vaginal bleeding between menstrual periods) may be the first sign of cervical cancer.   (M-S)

▶ When caring for a comatose client, the nurse should explain each step to the client in a normal voice.   (M-S)

▶ A client who's receiving phenytoin (Dilantin) is at risk for gingival hyperplasia.
                                                                            (M-S)

▶ When providing denture care, the nurse should line the sink with a washcloth or a paper towel to prevent breakage if the dentures are dropped.   (M-S)

▶ The client should void within 6 to 8 hours after surgery.   (M-S)

▶ EEG readings identify normal and abnormal brain waves.   (M-S)

▶ Migraine headaches cause persistent, severe pain, usually in the temporal region.   (M-S)

▶ A client who's in a bladder retraining program should void every 2 hours during the day and twice at night.   (M-S)

▶ The cardiovascular and respiratory systems are regulated by the autonomic nervous system.   (M-S)

▶ Ergotamine (Ergostat) is an effective treatment for migraine or vascular headaches.   (M-S)

▶ Signs and symptoms of hiatal hernia include fullness in the upper abdominal region, heartburn, and reflux.   (M-S)

▶ *Prophylaxis* is disease prevention.   (M-S)

▶ Women who have borne children have a higher incidence of cholelithiasis than any other group.   (M-S)

▶ Ascites and jaundice are prominent signs of advanced liver disease.   (M-S)

▶ *Obstipation* is protracted constipation or the absence of bowel movements.
                                                                        (M-S)

▶ Roasted chicken, rice, and pound cake are appropriate foods for a client on a low-residue diet.   (M-S)

▶ A rectal tube should remain in place for 20 to 30 minutes, and the client shouldn't get up after it has been inserted.   (M-S)

▶ Trust is the foundation of the nurse-client relationship.   (FND)

▶ In proper body alignment, the body parts are in correct relationship to their natural anatomical position.   (M-S)

▶ For the postoperative client, a diet high in carbohydrates and proteins is most therapeutic.   (M-S)

▶ *Blood pressure* is the pressure exerted on the arterial walls as blood is forced through them.   (FND)

▶ Clients who have hepatitis B should be instructed to never donate blood.
                                                                        (M-S)

▶ Clients who are undergoing radiation therapy should protect their skin markings because they are landmarks for treatment.   (M-S)

▶ Biopsy, with cytological examination of the tumor specimen, provides the most definitive diagnosis of cancer.   (M-S)

▶ Clients who are in methadone maintenance programs should receive methadone dissolved in 4 oz (118 ml) of orange juice or a powdered citrus drink unless the drug is provided in a liquid form.   (PSY)

▶ *Arthroplasty* is joint repair.   (M-S)

▶ When giving a client a bed bath, the nurse should follow this sequence: face, neck, arms, hands, chest, abdomen, back, legs, and perineum.   (FND)

▶ To avoid self-injury when lifting and moving a client, the nurse should use the large muscles of her thighs. **(FND)**

▶ A *sarcoma* is a malignant tumor of connective tissue. **(M-S)**

▶ *Subluxation* is partial dislocation of a joint. **(M-S)**

▶ Aluminum hydroxide (Amphojel) decreases gastric acidity. **(M-S)**

▶ Barbiturates may cause confusion and delirium in elderly clients who have organic brain disorders. **(PSY)**

▶ Physical therapy promotes optimal functioning in the client with arthritis. **(M-S)**

▶ Most clients who have hepatitis A are anicteric (lacking jaundice). **(M-S)**

▶ Adding a toe pleat to the top sheet makes a client's feet more comfortable. **(FND)**

▶ Hepatitis A is highly contagious during the preicteric phase. **(M-S)**

▶ The nurse must follow standard precautions when caring for a client who has hepatitis A. **(M-S)**

▶ Cholecystography isn't effective in diagnosing gallstones. The stones may obstruct the cystic duct and prevent the contrast medium from entering the gallbladder. **(M-S)**

▶ *Anticipatory grief* is grief that arises in anticipation of an inevitable death or a significant loss. **(M-S)**

▶ Because of polyuria, dehydration is a major concern for clients who have diabetes insipidus. **(M-S)**

▶ To guard against a charge of malpractice, the nurse should provide care in a reasonable and prudent manner according to accepted standards of care. **(FND)**

▶ The client may receive methohexital (Brevital), a general anesthetic, before electroconvulsive therapy. **(PSY)**

▶ When caring for a client who's receiving electroconvulsive therapy, maintaining a patent airway is the nurse's highest priority. **(PSY)**

▶ The decision to use restraints on a client must be based on safety and the needs of the client. **(M-S)**

▶ The physician may prescribe diphenhydramine (Benadryl) to relieve extrapyramidal adverse reactions of psychotropic medications. **(PSY)**

▶ A client whose condition is stabilized with lithium should have blood drug levels drawn every month. **(PSY)**

▶ To prevent "purple glove" syndrome, the nurse shouldn't administer phenytoin I.V. through a vein in the back of the client's hand. **(M-S)**

▶ Psychotropic medications are used to relieve symptoms and allow the client to participate in therapy.   (PSY)

▶ Through behavior, the manipulative client is asking to be controlled.   (PSY)

▶ A client who has signs or symptoms of lithium toxicity should be instructed not to take any additional doses and should be examined by a physician.
                                                                              (PSY)

▶ Alcoholics Anonymous teaches members that alcoholism is progressive.
                                                                              (PSY)

▶ Methylphenidate (Ritalin) is the drug of choice for children who have attention deficit hyperactivity disorder.   (PED)

▶ Setting consistent limits is the most effective way to control a client's manipulative behavior.   (PSY)

▶ Violent outbursts are common in clients who have borderline personality disorder.   (PSY)

▶ When caring for a depressed client, the nurse should explore meaningful losses.
                                                                              (PSY)

▶ An *illusion* is a false interpretation of a sensory stimulus.   (PSY)

▶ Extrapyramidal adverse reactions are common in clients who take antipsychotic medications.   (PSY)

▶ *Anxiety* is a vague sense of impending doom or apprehension without real cause.   (PSY)

▶ The signs and symptoms of Cushing's syndrome result primarily from unregulated secretion of glucocorticoids and androgens.   (M-S)

▶ *Confabulation* is a speech pattern and is the unconscious filling in of memory gaps with fabricated information. It occurs in Korsakoff's syndrome.   (PSY)

▶ The goal of any therapy is to bring about a positive change.   (PSY)

▶ *Catharsis* is the therapeutic release of pent-up feelings and emotions by open discussion of ideas and thoughts.   (PSY)

▶ A basic assumption of psychoanalytic theory is that all behavior has a cause and can be explained.   (PSY)

▶ Total parenteral nutrition solutions contain glucose, amino acids, and electrolytes.   (M-S)

▶ Regional anesthesia may involve the use of topical anesthetics, local infiltration, nerve blocks, or subdural or epidural blocks.   (M-S)

▶ Children between ages 2 and 3 discover masturbation as an enjoyable activity while exploring their bodies.   (PED)

▶ Respiratory paralysis occurs during stage IV of general anesthesia.   **(M-S)**

▶ The nurse should encourage ambulation in the postpartum client who has gas pains and flatulence.   **(MAT)**

▶ After delivery of the placenta, uterine massage helps to stimulate contractions.   **(MAT)**

▶ During phototherapy, the nurse should cover the infant's eyes to prevent retinal injury.   **(MAT)**

▶ Crackles indicate lung congestion caused by fluid or pus.   **(M-S)**

▶ Bronchovesicular breath sounds are abnormal when heard over the peripheral lung fields.   **(M-S)**

▶ Wheezing is an abnormal, high-pitched breath sound that indicates obstruction or closure of the bronchi.   **(FND)**

▶ The nurse should use mineral oil to remove an insect from the client's external ear canal.   **(M-S)**

▶ If a client complains that his hearing aid isn't working, the nurse should first check the switch and batteries.   **(M-S)**

▶ The nurse should grade hyperactive deep tendon reflexes with sustained clonus as +4.   **(FND)**

▶ Vertigo is the major assessment finding in a client who has Ménière's disease.   **(M-S)**

▶ The nurse should instruct the client who has an upper respiratory infection to blow his nose with both nostrils open.   **(M-S)**

▶ An infant who has gastroesophageal reflux should receive formula thickened with cereal.   **(PED)**

▶ A client can resume most normal activities 3 or 4 days after cataract surgery.   **(M-S)**

▶ Ocular irritation, a decreasing visual field, corneal edema, and scleral redness are signs of corneal transplant graft rejection.   **(M-S)**

▶ A child should visit the dentist by age 2.   **(PED)**

▶ Wisdom teeth usually appear between ages 17 and 21.   **(PED)**

▶ Signs and symptoms of Graves' disease include nervousness, irritability, weight loss, palpitations, increased thirst, and exophthalmos.   **(M-S)**

▶ When caring for a postoperative client who's allowed to have oral intake, the nurse should force fluids to help prevent constipation.   **(M-S)**

▶ Preschoolers don't view death as final, but fear separation from their parents.   **(PED)**

▶ Infection can be transmitted through saliva, feces, urine, vomitus, and blood, and through nasal, penile, and vaginal discharge. **(M-S)**

▶ Breech presentation of the fetus increases the risk of prolapsed umbilical cord, fetal head trauma, and fracture of the fetal spine or arm. **(MAT)**

▶ A nasal cannula delivers oxygen concentrations of 22% to 44%. **(M-S)**

▶ Postmenopausal women who receive estrogen replacement therapy are at increased risk for gallbladder disease. **(M-S)**

▶ The hormone oxytocin stimulates powerful uterine contractions during labor. **(MAT)**

▶ Prolactin stimulates the production of breast milk. **(MAT)**

▶ Polyuria and polyphagia are signs of diabetes insipidus. **(M-S)**

▶ A client who has diabetic ketoacidosis experiences osmotic diuresis that leads to dehydration and electrolyte loss. **(M-S)**

▶ Cushing's syndrome causes moon face, buffalo hump, acne, mood swings, hirsutism, amenorrhea, and decreased libido. **(M-S)**

▶ In group therapy, each member of the group has the opportunity to examine interactions, learn and practice successful interpersonal communication skills, and explore emotional conflicts. **(PSY)**

▶ Signs of nasal fracture include internal and external bleeding, swelling of adjacent soft tissues, and deformity. **(M-S)**

▶ When caring for a client with heart failure, the nurse should elevate the head of the bed. **(M-S)**

▶ Lip cancer causes a painless, indurated ulcer with raised edges. **(M-S)**

▶ The client whose signs and symptoms suggest stroke should be positioned on the affected side. **(M-S)**

▶ After chest surgery, the nurse should encourage the client to raise the arm on the affected side above the head frequently. **(M-S)**

▶ Variable decelerations of the fetal heart rate indicates compression or prolapse of the umbilical cord. **(MAT)**

▶ By age 4 months, infants have developed hand–eye coordination. **(PED)**

▶ The nurse should withhold all preparations that contain vitamin D from the client who's receiving calcifediol (Calderol). **(M-S)**

▶ In a client who's receiving digoxin, a below-normal serum potassium level increases the risk of digoxin toxicity. **(M-S)**

▶ A client who has diabetes insipidus may crave cold water. **(M-S)**

▶ Flurazepam (Dalmane) toxicity causes mental confusion, hallucinations, and ataxia. (M-S)

▶ A "silent" myocardial infarction causes no symptoms and is detected on an electrocardiogram. (M-S)

▶ Adverse effects of verapamil (Calan) include dizziness, headache, constipation, hypotension, and atrioventricular conduction disturbances. (M-S)

▶ Yellowish-green wound drainage indicates an infection. (M-S)

▶ During a sickle cell crisis, severe pain in the hands and feet is known as "hand-foot" syndrome. (M-S)

▶ Oral candidiasis causes white plaques with a milk-curd appearance on the oral mucosa, gums, or tongue. (M-S)

▶ A client who has paranoid personality disorder shows pervasive, long-standing suspicions that reflect a lack of basic trust. (PSY)

▶ A person who has antisocial personality disorder perceives others and the world in general as hostile and harmful. (PSY)

▶ Failing to provide a safe, secure environment for a child is child neglect. (FND)

▶ The most common psychiatric disorder is depression. (PSY)

▶ Cytomegalovirus, a member of the herpesvirus family, can cause extensive fetal damage. (MAT)

▶ Infants with cerebral palsy may have asymmetrical movements, difficulty feeding, and excessive or feeble crying. (PED)

▶ Anorexia, weight loss, abdominal pain, and jaundice may be the first signs and symptoms of pancreatic cancer. (M-S)

▶ Adverse effects of tricyclic antidepressant drugs include tachycardia and orthostatic hypotension. (PSY)

▶ Tocolytic therapy is usually indicated for the client who's in premature labor. (MAT)

▶ *Snow blindness* is temporary dimming of vision caused by the glare of the sun on snow. (M-S)

▶ Hodgkin's disease characteristically causes painless, progressive enlargement of lymph nodes. (M-S)

▶ In Huntington's chorea, degeneration of the cerebral cortex and basal ganglia causes progressive dyskinetic movements and mental deterioration. (M-S)

▶ The nurse should stay alert for suicidal behavior in clients with Huntington's chorea. (M-S)

▶ Foods high in vitamin D include fortified milk, fish (especially herring), liver, liver oil, and egg yolk. **(M-S)**

▶ For a pelvic examination, the nurse should place the client in the lithotomy position. If the client can't assume a lithotomy position (for example, because of advanced age or poor health), the nurse should place the client on her left side. **(M-S)**

▶ During a vaginal examination, an assistant should be present regardless of the sex of the examiner. **(M-S)**

▶ Before ovulation, the cervical mucus is thick and doesn't stretch when pulled between the thumb and finger. **(M-S)**

▶ Discoloration of body fluids is a common adverse effect of rifampin (Rimactane). **(M-S)**

▶ Liver function tests should be performed before a client starts isoniazid (INH) therapy. **(M-S)**

▶ Bread and cereal are good sources of thiamine, iron, niacin, and riboflavin. **(M-S)**

▶ Central cyanosis is the most significant sign of hypoxia. **(M-S)**

▶ Good Samaritan laws protect health care professionals who provide assistance at the scene of an emergency without fear of a lawsuit arising from such assistance. **(FND)**

▶ Within 24 hours, the physician should sign medical orders given verbally or by telephone. **(FND)**

▶ The nurse should refer the client's questions about informed consent to the physician. **(FND)**

▶ A competent adult has the right to refuse life-saving medical treatment; however, the client must be fully informed of the consequences of refusal. **(FND)**

▶ An intoxicated client isn't considered competent to refuse required medical treatment. **(FND)**

▶ The client's health record or chart is the hospital's physical property; however, the contents belong to the client. **(FND)**

▶ The client or legal guardian must give written consent before the client's records can be released to a third party. **(FND)**

▶ The nurse can't perform duties that violate a rule or regulation established by a state licensing board, no matter who orders those duties. **(FND)**

▶ When caring for a client who's hostile or angry, the nurse should try to remain calm and continue to listen impartially. **(FND)**

▶ When caring for a sick or injured child who has limited communication skills, the nurse may encourage the child to draw pictures to express his feelings.   (PED)

▶ To conduct a health history interview, the nurse should choose a private room, preferably one with a door that can be closed.   (FND)

▶ When caring for an acutely ill or agitated client, the nurse should limit questions to those that can provide essential information.   (FND)

▶ Before taking an oral temperature, the nurse should wait 15 minutes after the client has smoked a cigarette or taken anything by mouth.   (FND)

▶ The nurse shouldn't use her thumb to take the client's pulse.   (FND)

▶ When counting respirations, the nurse should count an inspiration and an expiration as one respiration.   (FND)

▶ *Kussmaul's respiration* is a breathing pattern in which respirations are abnormally fast and deep and aren't separated by pauses.   (FND)

▶ In *Cheyne-Stokes respiration*, periods of deep, rapid breathing alternate with periods of apnea.   (FND)

▶ *Eupnea* is normal respiration.   (FND)

▶ Biot's respiration is characterized by periods of apnea alternating with periods in which the client takes four or five breaths of identical depth.   (FND)

▶ Before thyroid surgery, clients with hyperthyroidism usually receive potassium iodine to reduce the size and vascularity of the goiter.   (M-S)

▶ When taking blood pressure, the nurse should support the client's arm rather than letting the client use his own strength to hold his arm up.   (FND)

▶ Nonmodifiable risk factors for coronary artery disease include heredity, sex, race, and age.   (M-S)

▶ Inspection is the most common assessment technique.   (FND)

▶ The nurse should instruct the pregnant vegetarian client to obtain adequate protein from nonmeat sources.   (MAT)

▶ The pregnant client should take only prescribed prenatal vitamins and should avoid high-potency, over-the-counter megavitamin preparations.   (MAT)

▶ Foods that are high in sodium can cause fluid retention.   (M-S)

▶ Adding fiber to the diet can help the pregnant client avoid constipation and hemorrhoids.   (M-S)

▶ The normal life cycle of a red blood cell is 120 days.   (M-S)

▶ Ritualism is a typical behavior in a toddler.   (PED)

▶ A person with 20/100 vision sees at 20' (6.1 m) what a person with normal vision sees at 100' (30.5 m). **(M-S)**

▶ According to Freud's psychosexual theory, the oral stage occurs from birth to age 18 months. **(PED)**

▶ Food interferes with the absorption of penicillin. **(M-S)**

▶ Offering a favorite "chaser," such as orange juice, is one way to encourage a child to swallow oral medication. **(PED)**

▶ To provide a comfortable atmosphere, the nurse should advise family members to take some personal items when moving the client to a skilled nursing facility. **(FND)**

▶ When prioritizing nursing diagnoses, the nurse should give life-threatening problems top priority. **(FND)**

▶ When developing a nursing care plan, the nurse should write client outcomes in measurable, observable terms and include target dates for their completion. The acronym *SMART* means specific, measurable, achievable, reasonable, and time factor. **(FND)**

▶ *Spinal shock* is loss of all spinal reflexes and sensations below the level of injury after spinal cord transection. **(M-S)**

▶ When inserting a nasogastric tube, the nurse should aim the tube downward and toward the ear that's closer to the nostril that's being used. **(M-S)**

▶ The nurse should inform the client who's taking oral iron (ferrous sulfate) that the preparation may turn his feces dark green to black. **(M-S)**

▶ Polycythemia vera causes pruritus, pain in the fingers and toes, hyperuricemia, a florid complexion, weakness, and easy fatigue. **(M-S)**

▶ Rheumatic fever is usually preceded by a group A beta-hemolytic streptococcal infection. **(M-S)**

▶ *Thyroid storm* is a medical crisis caused by uncontrolled hyperthyroidism and characterized by hyperpyrexia and tachycardia. **(M-S)**

▶ Tardive dyskinesia causes involuntary repetitive movements of the face and mouth, such as lip smacking, and can progress to other abnormal movements. **(M-S)**

▶ Vision is usually fully developed by age 7. **(PED)**

▶ The nurse shouldn't give raisins, hot dogs, or round foods, such as grapes, to an infant because these foods may cause choking. **(PED)**

▶ Hydrocephalus is the most common complication of surgical closure of a myelomeningocele. **(PED)**

▶ In a client with hemophilia, repeated hemorrhages may cause degenerative joint changes, osteoporosis, and muscle atrophy.   (M-S)

▶ For the child who has failure to thrive, the goal of care is to promote an age-appropriate pattern of growth and development.   (PED)

▶ A client who has mania should avoid competitive games, heated group discussions, and excessive physical exercise.   (PSY)

▶ After thyroidectomy, a hoarse or whispery voice suggests damage to the laryngeal nerves.   (M-S)

▶ After intracranial surgery, the nurse should keep the client in a lateral or semi-prone position until consciousness returns.   (M-S)

▶ During the immediate postoperative period after intracranial surgery, the nurse should monitor the client's vital signs and assess his level of consciousness for signs of increasing intracranial pressure.   (M-S)

▶ Techniques used in chest physiotherapy include percussion (patting the back with cupped hands) and vibration (placing the hands over the affected area and vigorously quivering them).   (M-S)

▶ Folic acid and vitamin B_{12} are essential for nucleoprotein synthesis and red blood cell maturation.   (M-S)

▶ The nurse should encourage the parents of a hearing-impaired child to communicate through mime, gestures, and body language.   (PED)

▶ Clients who are receiving prednisone should consume a high-protein, high-potassium, low-salt diet.   (M-S)

▶ As a general rule, neonates require 120 cal/kg of body weight at birth.   (MAT)

▶ Physical abuse of a child is suggested by a parent's implausible explanation of how the child's injuries occurred.   (PED)

▶ In geriatric clients, age-related changes and multiple medications contribute to a high incidence of noncompliance with drug therapy.   (M-S)

▶ Strawberry tongue is a sign of Kawasaki's disease.   (M-S)

▶ A first-degree burn involves the stratum corneum, the outermost layer of the skin; it causes pain and reddened skin.   (M-S)

▶ A client who's being treated for an asthma attack should be placed in the semi-Fowler or high Fowler position, depending on the client's comfort.   (M-S)

▶ Tuberculosis is a reportable communicable disease that's caused by *Mycobacterium tuberculosis*, an acid-fast bacillus.   (M-S)

▶ In right-sided cardiac catheterization, a radiopaque catheter passes through the antecubital or femoral vein and into the client's right atrium, right ventricle, and pulmonary vasculature. **(M-S)**

▶ The average length of the menstruation cycle is 28 days. **(M-S)**

▶ McDonald's rule is used to measure fundal height to determine the length of pregnancy. **(MAT)**

▶ Nägele's rule (subtract 3 months from the first day of the last menstrual period and then add 7 days) is used to calculate the expected date of delivery. **(MAT)**

▶ *Amenorrhea* is a presumptive sign of pregnancy. **(MAT)**

▶ The nurse should inform the pregnant client that oral sex during pregnancy may cause air embolism. **(MAT)**

▶ Human chorionic gonadotropin in the blood or urine is a probable sign of pregnancy. **(MAT)**

▶ The pregnant woman should avoid exposure to X-rays, especially during the first trimester. **(MAT)**

▶ Sexual intercourse during pregnancy is contraindicated if the amniotic membranes have ruptured or if vaginal bleeding has occurred. **(MAT)**

▶ Milia are small papules that are sometimes seen on the cheek or the bridge of the nose in neonates. **(MAT)**

▶ The union of the male and female gametes results in a zygote. **(MAT)**

▶ In a stroke, blood vessels in the brain are blocked by an embolus or a hemorrhage. As a result, blood supply is decreased to brain tissues that are normally perfused by the damaged vessels. **(M-S)**

▶ After a fracture, bone healing occurs in the following sequence: inflammation, cellular proliferation, callus formation, ossification, and remodeling. **(M-S)**

▶ The nurse shouldn't give atropine to a client who has glaucoma. **(M-S)**

▶ Once the zygote is implanted in the uterus, it is called an embryo. **(FND)**

▶ Fetal growth occurs in a cephalocaudal fashion. **(FND)**

▶ The pons is located in front of the cerebellum, between the midbrain and the medulla. **(M-S)**

▶ Smooth muscles are controlled by the autonomic nervous system. **(M-S)**

▶ Flexion contractures of the hips may develop in a client who's wheelchair bound. **(M-S)**

▶ Immediate care for a sprain or strain consists of applying ice and elevating the limb above the level of the client's heart. **(M-S)**

▶ According to Erikson, the main conflict of the young adult (ages 19 to 35) is intimacy versus isolation. **(FND)**

▶ Erikson proposed that the main conflict of the older adult (age 65 and older) is integrity versus despair. **(FND)**

▶ Family therapy focuses on the family as a whole rather than on an individual member. **(PSY)**

▶ The erythrocyte sedimentation rate for women is normally 0 to 20 mm/hour. **(M-S)**

▶ The erythrocyte sedimentation rate for men is normally 0 to 10 mm/hour. **(M-S)**

▶ In culdoscopy, the physician visualizes the pelvic organs with an endoscope inserted through the posterior vaginal wall. **(M-S)**

▶ Propranolol (Inderal) blocks the sympathetic nerve stimulation that increases the cardiac workload during exercise or stress. **(M-S)**

▶ Electrocardiogram (ECG) changes usually appear during the first 24 hours after a myocardial infarction, but in some cases, they are delayed for 5 to 6 days. **(M-S)**

▶ Cottage cheese, fish, canned beans, chuck steak, chocolate pudding, Italian salad dressing, dill pickles, and beef broth are extremely high in sodium. **(M-S)**

▶ Prunes, watermelons, dried lima beans, soybeans, bananas, oranges, nectarines, and cantaloupes are high in potassium. **(M-S)**

▶ The neonate of a diabetic mother should be assessed for hypoglycemia. **(MAT)**

▶ A client who has delivered a stillborn child should be allowed to hold the child to help her come to terms with the death. **(MAT)**

▶ The concept of *object permanence* (knowing that something still exists when it's out of view) develops between ages 6 months and 10 months. **(PED)**

▶ During the sensorimotor stage, a child begins to learn about cause-and-effect relationships. **(PED)**

▶ According to Erikson, a conscience begins to develop during the preschool years (ages 3 to 6). **(FND)**

▶ *Molding* is shaping of the fetal head as it adjusts to the shape and size of the birth canal. **(MAT)**

▶ Liver dysfunction may cause difficulty metabolizing certain drugs, resulting in toxicity. **(M-S)**

▶ The nurse should monitor the client's blood pressure closely if a spinal block is administered before delivery. **(MAT)**

▶ If a client suddenly becomes hypotensive during labor, the nurse should increase the flow rate of I.V. fluids, as ordered, and turn the client on her side. **(MAT)**

▶ After delivery of the placenta, the nurse should anticipate adding oxytocin to the I.V. solution. **(MAT)**

▶ Early deceleration of the fetal heart rate is caused by compression of the fetal head during uterine contractions. No treatment is indicated. **(MAT)**

▶ Pregnant clients should take folic acid because this nutrient is essential for rapid cell division and the prevention of neural tube defects. **(MAT)**

▶ In such conditions as burns and malnutrition, edema is caused by a decrease in capillary osmotic pressure. **(M-S)**

▶ Fluid volume deficit is a potential complication of nasogastric suctioning. **(M-S)**

▶ Pulmonary congestion may lead to accumulation of fluid throughout the body. **(M-S)**

▶ A woman who has a spinal cord injury may still be able to become pregnant. **(M-S)**

▶ During the first few days after the onset of intracranial bleeding, nursing care should focus on providing a quiet, restful environment. **(M-S)**

▶ A client who's receiving clomiphene (Clomid) to induce ovulation should be told that this drug may cause multiple gestations. **(M-S)**

▶ Neurosyphilis is associated with a slapping gait and blindness. **(M-S)**

▶ Increasing intracranial pressure is the most serious complication of a stroke. **(M-S)**

▶ A pregnant client who has an incompetent cervix usually undergoes cervical suturing between weeks 14 and 18 to help her maintain the pregnancy. **(MAT)**

▶ To pinpoint the bleeding site in a client with an intracranial hemorrhage, the physician may order a cerebral arteriogram. **(M-S)**

▶ Factors that affect the action of drugs include drug absorption, distribution, metabolism, and excretion. **(M-S)**

▶ During the first trimester of pregnancy, the client should refrain from taking any drug unless lack of drug therapy would adversely affect her health. **(MAT)**

▶ Before a drug is prescribed to a woman of childbearing age, the physician should rule out the possibility of pregnancy. **(M-S)**

▶ Most drugs that are ingested by a lactating woman appear in the breast milk.
(MAT)

▶ Hemolytic anemia may develop when clients who have glucose-6-phosphate dehydrogenase deficiency are given sulfonamides. (M-S)

▶ Acidosis may cause insulin resistance. (M-S)

▶ The five pregnancy risk categories (A, B, C, D, and X) identify a drug's potential risk to the fetus. (M-S)

▶ The nurse should use the bell of the stethoscope to listen for venous hums and murmurs. (FND)

▶ The *chief complaint* is a subjective statement that's made by the client to describe his most significant needs and concerns. (FND)

▶ Turner's sign, or Grey Turner's sign, is seen in clients who have acute pancreatitis. (M-S)

▶ A client with a gastric ulcer typically has gnawing or burning epigastric pain. (M-S)

▶ To assess the client's general knowledge level, the nurse should ask questions such as, "Who is the president of the United States?" and other questions of general knowledge. (FND)

▶ The first cranial nerve is the olfactory nerve. (M-S)

▶ A client with cerebellar disease has an ataxic gait. (M-S)

▶ To check for cerebrospinal fluid leakage, the nurse should inspect the client's nose and ears for clear fluid. (M-S)

▶ Reye's syndrome is associated with the use of aspirin during certain viral illnesses such as chickenpox. (M-S)

▶ Compression syndrome occurs when pressure caused by edema pushes against encased arteries, veins, and nerves. (M-S)

▶ A client who has a ruptured ectopic pregnancy typically has sharp pain in the lower abdomen, spotting, and cramping. (MAT)

▶ The nurse should warn the client who's receiving prednisone or another steroid not to stop taking the drug abruptly. (M-S)

▶ Alanine aminotransferase and aspartate aminotransferase are liver enzymes. (M-S)

▶ The normal serum calcium level is 4.5 to 5.5 mEq/L. (M-S)

▶ The normal serum sodium level is 135 to 145 mEq/L. (M-S)

▶ The normal serum potassium level is 3.5 to 5.0 mEq/L. (M-S)

▶ A client who's receiving continuous ambulatory peritoneal dialysis must use sterile technique when performing catheter care.   **(M-S)**

▶ The Minnesota Multiphasic Personality Inventory is an objective test that assesses personality traits and characteristic ego responses to stress.   **(PSY)**

▶ The Stanford-Binet test assesses the intelligence and cognitive abilities of children younger than age 16.   **(PED)**

▶ T cells are involved in the cell-mediated immune response to microorganisms such as human immunodeficiency virus.   **(M-S)**

▶ For infants who are at high risk for acquired immunodeficiency syndrome, positive results on antibody tests are considered reliable after age 15 months.   **(PED)**

▶ When caring for a client who has acquired immunodeficiency syndrome, the nurse should wear a mask and protective eyewear if splashes of blood or other body fluids are likely to occur.   **(M-S)**

▶ The cardinal movements of labor are descent, flexion, internal rotation, extension, external rotation, and expulsion.   **(MAT)**

▶ Bence Jones protein is used to confirm the diagnosis of multiple myeloma (Hodgkin's disease).   **(M-S)**

▶ *Gaucher's disease* is an autosomal disorder characterized by abnormal accumulation of glucocerebrosides.   **(M-S)**

▶ A client with a colon obstruction usually has lower abdominal pain, constipation, increasing abdominal distention, and vomiting.   **(M-S)**

▶ Stools with the consistency of currant jelly are a sign of intussusception (telescoping of the intestine into itself).   **(M-S)**

▶ The tool used to diagnose a myocardial infarction is an electrocardiogram.   **(FND)**

▶ Allopurinol (Lopurin) is used to prevent or treat attacks of gout.   **(M-S)**

▶ Uric acid is an end product of purine metabolism.   **(M-S)**

▶ The normal sperm count is 120 to 300 million/ml.   **(M-S)**

▶ A man who has a sperm count of less than 60 million/ml is considered infertile.   **(M-S)**

▶ A pulsating abdominal mass indicates an aortic aneurysm.   **(M-S)**

▶ If the client's uterus is boggy after delivery of the placenta, the nurse should massage the fundus firmly.   **(MAT)**

▶ Passage of flatus and the return of bowel sounds indicate resumption of gastric motility.   **(M-S)**

▶ A person may use defense mechanisms to protect the ego during periods of anxiety. **(PSY)**

▶ *Projection* is an unconscious defense mechanism in which the person displaces generally negative feelings onto another individual. **(PSY)**

▶ *Displacement* is a defense mechanism in which the person transfers an emotion from its original object to a substitute. **(PSY)**

▶ The child with attention deficit hyperactivity disorder commonly has difficulty learning and staying focused. **(PSY)**

▶ A person who has agoraphobia is afraid of being alone or in a public area where escape would be difficult or help would be unavailable. **(PSY)**

▶ *Dementia* is a progressive organic mental disorder characterized by memory and intellectual deficits, disorientation, and decreased cognitive function. **(PSY)**

▶ The white blood cell count is normally 4,000 to 10,000/µl. **(M-S)**

▶ Serum cholesterol levels of 200 to 320 mg/dl are considered elevated. **(M-S)**

▶ Serum thyroxine (T_4) levels are normally 5 to 13.5 mcg/dl. **(M-S)**

▶ Production of human chorionic gonadotropin peaks around the 10th week of gestation. **(MAT)**

▶ Port-wine–colored amniotic fluid may indicate abruptio placentae. **(MAT)**

▶ A lecithin–sphingomyelin ratio of greater than 2:1 indicates fetal lung maturity. **(MAT)**

▶ Chorionic villi sampling is used to detect fetal chromosomal abnormalities. **(MAT)**

▶ Cloudy cerebrospinal fluid indicates infection. **(M-S)**

▶ During a lumbar puncture, crying, coughing, or straining may increase the amount of cerebrospinal fluid obtained. **(M-S)**

▶ To determine how far to insert a nasogastric tube, the nurse should measure the distance from the tip of the client's nose to the earlobe and add this measurement to the measured distance from the earlobe to the base of the xiphoid process. **(FND)**

▶ After colonoscopy, signs and symptoms of bowel perforation include malaise, rectal bleeding, abdominal pain and distention, fever, and mucopurulent drainage. **(M-S)**

▶ A *tort* is a wrongful act committed outside of a contractual relationship. Examples include battery (such as administering a drug over a client's objections) and assault (such as threatening a client with an injection if he refuses oral medication). **(FND)**

▶ *Slander* is a false and defamatory oral statement about a person.   (FND)

▶ Careful, accurate, and complete documentation is the nurse's best protection against a lawsuit.   (FND)

▶ According to Maslow's hierarchy of needs, physiologic needs are the most basic, followed in descending order by safety and security, belonging and affection, esteem and self-respect, and self-actualization.   (FND)

▶ According to Maslow, primary needs must be met to maintain life; secondary needs must be met to maintain the quality of life.   (FND)

▶ The *deciduous teeth* are the first teeth.   (PED)

▶ Abstinence is the only method that's 100% effective in preventing pregnancy and sexually transmitted diseases.   (M-S)

▶ The mother can nurse the neonate immediately after birth.   (MAT)

▶ Dopamine (Intropin) is the drug of choice for treating cardiogenic shock. It improves myocardial contractility and blood flow.   (M-S)

▶ Cranial nerve II (the optic nerve) is a sensory nerve that's responsible for vision.   (M-S)

▶ A client who has schizophrenia commonly has an absent, flat, blunted, or inappropriate affect.   (PSY)

▶ Crisis intervention focuses only on the client's immediate problems.   (PSY)

▶ In health care, *quality assurance* is evaluation of the services provided and the results achieved compared with accepted standards. This evaluation typically includes the quality, quantity, appropriateness, and costs of the health services provided.   (FND)

▶ All clients have the right to considerate and respectful care.   (FND)

▶ *Beneficence* is the quality or state of producing good, such as performing acts of charity or kindness.   (FND)

▶ The geriatric client normally has decreased bladder capacity and a delayed voiding sensation.   (M-S)

▶ The serum glucose level is normally 70 to 110 mg/dl.   (M-S)

▶ Lactated Ringer's solution is an isotonic solution.   (M-S)

▶ A serum sodium level of less than 135 mEq/L indicates hyponatremia. (M-S)

▶ The nurse shouldn't use a cotton-tipped applicator to dry the client's ear canal or to remove wax.   (FND)

▶ The nurse should instruct the client with a history of heat stroke to wear loose-fitting clothing, rest frequently, and drink plenty of fluids when exposed to extreme heat.   (FND)

▶ All central venous catheter ports should be capped when not in use. (M-S)

▶ Signs and symptoms of premenstrual syndrome include abdominal distention, engorged and painful breasts, backache, headache, and irritability. (M-S)

▶ Hip fracture is the most common fracture in geriatric clients and typically results from a fall. (M-S)

▶ During continuous tube feeding, the nurse should irrigate the tube every 6 hours. (M-S)

▶ The GI tract isn't sterile. (M-S)

▶ In an adult, hypothyroidism may cause coarse, dry hair with patchy loss or thinning. (M-S)

▶ A hair comb should have dull teeth. Sharp teeth could injure the client. (FND)

▶ Ligation and stripping of a vein is one treatment for varicosities. (M-S)

▶ Tepid water is 80° to 98° F (27° to 37° C). (FND)

▶ When using a heat lamp, the nurse should direct the lamp to the side of the treatment area, not directly over it. (FND)

▶ Foods that become liquid at room temperature or break down into liquid in the GI tract, such as ice cream, must be charted as fluid intake. (FND)

▶ Pulmonary edema can develop in minutes and results when fluid shifts from the vascular to the interstitial alveoli. (M-S)

▶ The nurse should administer routine medications within 30 minutes of the ordered time. (FND)

▶ Heparin is the drug of choice to treat thromboembolic disease. (M-S)

▶ The surgeon can use a Fogarty embolectomy catheter to extract an embolus from a large artery. (M-S)

▶ Blockage of a large artery by an embolus is a life-threatening emergency that requires immediate surgery. (M-S)

▶ Acute iliofemoral venous thrombosis causes limb enlargement. It can be detected by measuring the affected part and comparing it with the opposite extremity. (M-S)

▶ The areas that sustain the greatest damage from arteriosclerosis are the brain, heart, GI tract, kidneys, and extremities. (M-S)

▶ The nurse should inform a client who's receiving phenazopyridine (Pyridium) that this drug colors the urine orange or red. (M-S)

▶ To obtain a child's rectal temperature, the nurse should insert the thermometer only 1″ (2.5 cm) into the rectum. (PED)

▶ Normally, a neonate's urine specific gravity is 1.002 to 1.010 after ingesting milk. **(PED)**

▶ Laboratory test results are considered objective data. **(FND)**

▶ *Pneumocystis carinii* pneumonia usually causes disease only in people with suppressed immune systems. **(M-S)**

▶ For best absorption, clients should take erythromycin tablets with a full glass of water 1 hour before or 2 hours after a meal. **(M-S)**

▶ Trismus is a sign of tetanus that involves the facial muscles. **(M-S)**

▶ Operating room nurses are usually held liable for failing to keep an accurate count of sponges and other items used in surgery. **(M-S)**

▶ Defense mechanisms protect the personality by reducing stress and anxiety. **(PSY)**

▶ *Suppression* is conscious inhibition of thoughts that provoke stress or anxiety. **(PSY)**

▶ Warfarin (Coumadin) is an oral anticoagulant. **(M-S)**

▶ Infants should be weighed and measured monthly until they're at least age 6 months. **(PED)**

▶ During the oral phase (the first 18 months), the infant derives satisfaction and pleasure from sucking and chewing. **(PED)**

▶ Infancy lasts from birth to age 12 months. **(PED)**

▶ The toddler stage starts at age 1 and ends at age 3. **(PED)**

▶ A client who's at risk for a pressure ulcer shouldn't be placed on a trochanter when the side-lying position is used. A 30-degree lateral position is recommended. **(FND)**

▶ Foods that are high in iron include organ meats such as liver, nuts, legumes, dried fruits, eggs, whole grains, fortified cereals, and green, leafy vegetables. **(FND)**

▶ The best sources of vitamin B_6 are liver, kidney, muscle meats, soybeans, corn, and whole-grain cereals. **(FND)**

▶ For a thoracentesis, the nurse should position the client upright. **(M-S)**

▶ Blood that's not transfused within 30 minutes after it's obtained should be returned to the blood bank. **(FND)**

▶ To administer a blood transfusion, the nurse should hang the blood bag about 36″ above the level of the client's heart. **(FND)**

▶ Gas bubbles and discoloration in a blood bag indicate bacterial growth. **(M-S)**

▶ Before transfusing a large amount of blood, the nurse should use a warming coil to warm it to a temperature of greater than 98.7° F (37° C).   (M-S)

▶ Initially, the neonate should breast-feed for 2 to 5 minutes at each breast and then progress gradually to breast-feeding for 10 or 15 minutes at each breast every 2 to 3 hours.   (MAT)

▶ To treat tender skin on the breasts or nipples, a breast-feeding woman should use only a mild emollient cream prescribed by the physician.   (MAT)

▶ Breast-feeding women should increase their daily fluid intake by 500 to 900 ml per day.   (MAT)

▶ The nurse should place the client who has a closed chest drainage system in the semi-Fowler position and encourage hourly coughing by manual splinting of the chest.   (M-S)

▶ In a one-bottle closed chest drainage system, the bottle acts as a water seal. The bottle provides suction and collects drainage and therefore shouldn't be emptied.   (M-S)

▶ In a two-bottle closed chest drainage system, the first bottle collects drainage and the second acts as a water seal and controls suction.   (M-S)

▶ In a three-bottle closed chest drainage system, the first bottle collects drainage, the second acts as a water seal, and the third controls suction.   (M-S)

▶ During colostomy irrigation, the nurse should hang the irrigating bag 18" to 20" (45.5 to 50.5 cm) above the stoma.   (M-S)

▶ The temperature of fluid used for colostomy irrigation shouldn't exceed 105° F (40.5° C).   (M-S)

▶ Signs of arterial obstruction caused by an embolism include absent pulse, anesthesia, paralysis, and pale, cool skin.   (M-S)

▶ Hyperventilation is associated with respiratory alkalosis.   (M-S)

▶ A mineral oil enema is contraindicated for clients with appendicitis, an acute surgical abdomen, fecal impaction, or intestinal obstruction.   (M-S)

▶ Psychodrama is used in group therapy to help participants gain new perceptions and self-awareness.   (PSY)

▶ A client who's admitted to a psychiatric hospital involuntarily doesn't have the right to sign out against medical advice (AMA).   (PSY)

▶ "People who live in glass houses shouldn't throw stones" and "A rolling stone gathers no moss" are examples of proverbs that may be used during a psychiatric interview to evaluate the client's abstract reasoning ability.   (PSY)

▶ Before carrying out a nursing procedure, the nurse should follow this rule: Always assess before action.   (FND)

▶ Case management nursing involves a case manager who plans and coordinates client care activities. **(FND)**

▶ Pinpoint pupils are a sign of acute opioid intoxication. **(M-S)**

▶ The nursing history consists primarily of subjective assessment data. **(FND)**

▶ The physical examination provides objective assessment data obtained using the senses. **(FND)**

▶ The nurse gathers objective assessment data through inspection, percussion, palpation, and auscultation. **(FND)**

▶ Diagnostic test results provide objective assessment data. **(FND)**

▶ The client's toenails can be cleaned with an orangewood stick while his foot is immersed in water. **(FND)**

▶ A complete nursing diagnosis includes the client problem, the etiology (cause or contributing factor) of the problem, and signs or symptoms to help clarify the nursing diagnosis. **(FND)**

▶ The client's nails should be clipped and filed straight across, even with the end of the digit (what's called the *fat pad*). **(FND)**

▶ Antibiotics are used to reduce inflammation in diverticulitis. **(M-S)**

▶ Signs and symptoms of acute barbiturate intoxication may resemble those of alcohol intoxication. **(M-S)**

▶ A *labile affect* is characterized by a rapid shift of emotions and mood. **(PSY)**

▶ *Amnesia* is memory loss that results from an organic or inorganic cause. **(PSY)**

▶ Borderline personality disorder is marked by pervasive instability of self-image, mood, and interpersonal relationships. **(PSY)**

▶ Decreased renal function makes geriatric clients more susceptible to dehydration. **(M-S)**

▶ When giving an I.M. injection to an elderly client, the nurse should use a shorter needle. **(FND)**

▶ *Stress incontinence* is intermittent leakage of urine caused by a sudden increase in intra-abdominal pressure, such as from coughing, laughing, or running. **(M-S)**

▶ Gallstones may cause acute pancreatitis. **(M-S)**

▶ A client who's in restraints should be checked every 15 to 30 minutes, and each restraint should be removed every 2 hours. **(FND)**

▶ A client who's taking disulfiram (Antabuse) shouldn't receive metronidazole (Flagyl) because the drugs may interact to cause a psychotic reaction. **(M-S)**

▶ *Urge incontinence* is the inability to control a sudden urge to urinate.   (M-S)

▶ *Total incontinence* is continued urine leakage.   (M-S)

▶ Elderly people are often constipated because they have reduced intestinal motility.   (M-S)

▶ Protein, vitamin, and mineral needs usually remain constant as a person ages.   (FND)

▶ The elderly client becomes shorter as intervertebral spaces narrow and spinal curvature increases.   (M-S)

▶ When converting grams to grains, the nurse should remember the following rule: 1 g = 1,000 mg = 15 gr.   (FND)

▶ Before a client gives informed consent, he must receive information that would affect a reasonable person's decision to consent to or refuse a treatment or procedure. This information includes a description of the treatment or procedure, its potential risks and adverse effects, and the possible effects of refusing the treatment or procedure.   (FND)

▶ The client must sign a separate informed consent form for each treatment or procedure.   (FND)

▶ Gout progresses in four stages: asymptomatic hyperuricemia, acute gouty arthritis, intercritical gout, and chronic tophaceous gout.   (M-S)

▶ The nursing plan of care includes the nursing diagnosis, expected outcomes (or goals), nursing interventions, and evaluation criteria.   (FND)

▶ If the client received a sedative before signing an informed consent form, the nurse should notify the appropriate physician promptly.   (FND)

▶ During the acute phase of gout, the nurse should use a bed cradle to raise the sheets and blankets off of the client's sensitive joints.   (M-S)

▶ Congenital hip dysplasia is the most common hip joint disorder in children younger than age 3.   (PED)

▶ Heparin inactivates thromboplastin and thrombin.   (M-S)

▶ Placing a familiar object or picture on a door may assist a confused client to find his room without help.   (PSY)

▶ A client is demonstrating autonomy when he makes simple decisions, such as what time to take a bath.   (M-S)

▶ For the client with traction pins, the main purpose of skin care is to prevent infection.   (M-S)

▶ A client who's receiving morphine shouldn't take anticholinesterase agents. The resulting drug interaction may cause respiratory depression.   (M-S)

▶ Purulent drainage from a wound indicates the development of infection and delayed wound healing. **(M-S)**

▶ *Reframing* provides the client with alternative ways to view a situation. **(PSY)**

▶ In the early stage of Alzheimer's disease, short-term memory loss occurs. **(PSY)**

▶ Profound changes in personal relationships occur during the middle and advanced stages of Alzheimer's disease. **(PSY)**

▶ During the final stage of Alzheimer's disease, total memory loss occurs. **(PSY)**

▶ The nurse should wash her hands with warm, not hot, water. Warm water removes fewer protective skin oils. **(FND)**

▶ The cause of essential hypertension is unknown. **(M-S)**

▶ Administration of propranolol (Inderal) reduces portal pressure and decreases the risk of bleeding from esophageal varices. **(M-S)**

▶ The nurse should administer sedatives cautiously to a client with cirrhosis. **(M-S)**

▶ A client who has a burn wound that's infected with *Staphylococcus aureus* must be kept in strict isolation. **(M-S)**

▶ A client who's undergoing external radiation therapy should be instructed to avoid applying creams or lotions to the treatment site. **(M-S)**

▶ Strabismus is a normal finding in the neonate. **(MAT)**

▶ The most common vascular complication of diabetes mellitus is atherosclerosis. **(M-S)**

▶ Insulin deficiency may lead to hyperglycemia. **(M-S)**

▶ Drooling, a masklike expression, pill rolling, and a propulsive gait are signs of Parkinson's disease. **(M-S)**

▶ The point of maximal impulse is located at the fifth intercostal space, near the apex of the heart. **(FND)**

▶ The first heart sound (S_1) represents closure of the mitral and tricuspid valves. **(FND)**

▶ The second heart sound (S_2) represents closure of the aortic and pulmonic valves. **(FND)**

▶ Threatening a client with an injection for failing to take an oral medication is considered assault. **(FND)**

▶ The coronary artery supplies blood to the myocardium. **(M-S)**

▶ A client who has gouty arthritis should increase his fluid intake to prevent the formation of renal calculi. **(M-S)**

▶ The nurse should instruct a client who's following a low-salt diet to avoid canned vegetables. **(FND)**

▶ A client who's taking furosemide (Lasix) should eat bananas and citrus fruits because they're a good source of potassium. **(M-S)**

▶ Dyspnea is a common sign of left ventricular failure. **(M-S)**

▶ The nurse should encourage the client who is at risk for pneumonia to turn frequently, cough, and breathe deeply. **(M-S)**

▶ If the client's blood pressure rises 30 mm Hg above the baseline value, the nurse should notify the physician. **(FND)**

▶ In the client with a fractured hip, Buck's traction is used to immobilize and reduce spasms before surgery. **(FND)**

▶ When caring for a client with a fractured hip, the nurse should check the neurovascular status of the extremities every 2 hours. **(M-S)**

▶ The nurse should use an abduction pillow or trochanter rolls to maintain abduction in the postoperative client who has a fractured hip. **(FND)**

▶ A fiberglass cast is more durable and dries more quickly than a plaster cast. **(M-S)**

▶ In the immobilized client, the most important circulatory complication to watch for is pulmonary embolism. **(M-S)**

▶ To relieve edema associated with an extremity fracture, the nurse should elevate the affected limb. **(M-S)**

▶ The treatment of choice for the client with osteomyelitis is I.V. antibiotics. **(M-S)**

▶ The postpartum client may resume sexual intercourse after the perineal and uterine wounds heal (usually 2 to 6 weeks after delivery). **(MAT)**

▶ A pregnant nurse shouldn't be assigned to work with a client who is infected with cytomegalovirus or has other contagious infections. **(MAT)**

▶ The nurse should suspect abuse if the client's wounds are inconsistent with the stated history or if the client has various wounds that are in different stages of healing. **(FND)**

▶ *Fetal demise* is the death of a fetus after the age of viability (20 weeks' gestation). **(MAT)**

▶ Administering oxytocin (Pitocin) is the most commonly used method to induce labor after artificial rupture of the membranes. **(MAT)**

▶ When caring for a terminally ill client, ensuring comfort is the nurse's highest priority. (M-S)

▶ The client who's prone to constipation should increase dietary bulk. (M-S)

▶ Dorsiflexion is recommended for immediate relief of leg cramps. (M-S)

▶ After cardiac surgery, the client should follow a diet that provides 2 g of sodium and 300 mg of cholesterol daily. (M-S)

▶ After the amniotic membranes rupture, the nurse's top priority is monitoring the fetal heart rate. (MAT)

▶ Bleeding after intercourse is an early sign of cervical cancer. (M-S)

▶ Oral hypoglycemics stimulate the secretion of insulin from the pancreatic islet cells. (M-S)

▶ Use of such drugs as antibiotics is a common cause of vaginal infections because they destroy the normal flora of the vagina. (M-S)

▶ The kidneys play a major role in maintaining the body's fluid balance. (M-S)

▶ People who visit a client who has a radiation implant must limit their stay to 10 minutes. (M-S)

▶ Reexamining one's goals is a major developmental task during middle adulthood. (FND)

▶ Docusate sodium (Colace) helps prevent straining during defecation. (M-S)

▶ Headache and restlessness are early indicators of delirium tremens. (PSY)

▶ According to most experts, the acute stage of alcohol detoxification encompasses the first 72 hours after consumption ends. (PSY)

▶ After prostatic surgery, the primary cause of pain is the indwelling urinary catheter. (M-S)

▶ A pregnant woman who has a cat is at increased risk for toxoplasmosis because the infecting organism (*Toxoplasma gondii*) is in cat feces. (MAT)

▶ *Telangiectatic nevi* (stork bites) are flat red or purple lesions that may appear on the nose, upper eyelids, or back of the neck of a neonate. (MAT)

▶ When assessing the neonate after a breech birth, the nurse should check for brachial nerve palsy. (MAT)

▶ Spontaneous abortion is a possible complication of amniocentesis. (MAT)

▶ If a pregnant client's urine tests positive for acetone but negative for glucose, her diet must be assessed for adequate protein intake. (MAT)

▶ During pregnancy, lack of exercise or a calcium deficiency may cause leg cramps. (MAT)

▶ Orange juice and green, leafy vegetables are good sources of folic acid. (FND)

▶ Exposure to rubella during pregnancy is associated with fetal heart defects and other anomalies. (MAT)

▶ When using the Glasgow Coma Scale, the nurse assesses the client's verbal response, motor response, and eye openings. (FND)

▶ During the first 24 hours after a major burn injury, the client should receive nothing by mouth and should receive I.V. fluid replacement according to the modified Brooke, Baxter, Parkland, or Evans formula. (M-S)

▶ The nurse should place an unconscious client in low Fowler's position when administering an intermittent nasogastric tube feeding. (M-S)

▶ *Decorticate positioning* is an abnormal posture in which the client's arms are adducted (toward the core of the body) and flexed, with the wrists and fingers flexed on the chest. (M-S)

▶ When caring for a client with drug-induced psychosis, the nurse should determine when the drug was taken. This information can help determine whether the drug can be eliminated from the body. (M-S)

▶ If a client's condition is likely to require surgery, he should be given nothing by mouth unless it's approved by the physician. (M-S)

▶ During the first trimester of pregnancy, increased hormonal levels may cause nausea and vomiting. (MAT)

▶ Morphine sulfate is used to relieve the pain of nephrolithiasis. (M-S)

▶ When caring for a client with thrombocytopenia, the nurse should institute measures to protect the client from injury. (M-S)

▶ As soon as possible after a client dies, the nurse should place the body in a normal position and close the client's eyes if they're open. (FND)

▶ Trendelenburg's test evaluates venous filling and is used to check for incompetent valves in a client who has varicose veins. (M-S)

▶ *Decerebrate positioning* is an abnormal posture in which the client's arms are adducted and extended, the wrists are pronated, the fingers are flexed, the legs are stiffly extended, and the feet are plantar flexed. (M-S)

▶ The best communication tool that the nurse can develop is effective listening. (FND)

▶ Cerebrospinal fluid is a transcellular fluid. (M-S)

▶ Sodium regulates extracellular osmolality. (M-S)

▶ In the early stages of shock, the heart and brain maintain blood circulation. (FND)

▶ Opioids may not effectively relieve phantom pain. (M-S)

▶ A trauma patient who has received multiple blood transfusions is at risk for hypocalcemia and hypothermia. (M-S)

▶ In a precipitous labor, delivery is unusually rapid, occurring only 2 hours after the onset of labor. (MAT)

▶ The nurse should advise the woman who's taking hormonal contraceptives not to smoke. (M-S)

▶ Cold constricts blood vessels on the body's surface. (FND)

▶ Giving a tepid sponge bath reduces the client's body temperature. (FND)

▶ When applying heat or cold, the nurse should take measures to protect the client from thermal injury. (FND)

▶ Application of moist heat warms the skin more quickly than dry heat. (FND)

▶ For a warm soak of an extremity, the water temperature shouldn't exceed 105° F (40.6° C). (FND)

▶ Infants and geriatric clients have reduced resistance to heat. (FND)

▶ After applying an ice pack, the nurse should discontinue the treatment if the client's skin becomes white or extremely red. (FND)

▶ Kernig's sign indicates meningitis. (M-S)

▶ Kernig's sign elicits both resistance and hamstring muscle pain when the examiner attempts to extend the knee while the hip and knee are both flexed 90 degrees. (M-S)

▶ A herniated nucleus pulposus (intervertebral disk) most commonly occurs in the lumbar and lumbosacral regions. (M-S)

▶ *Laminectomy* is surgical removal of a herniated portion of an intervertebral disk. (M-S)

▶ In the client who has a fractured and displaced femur, treatment starts with reduction and immobilization of the affected leg. (M-S)

▶ *Flight of ideas* is an altered thought process that's marked by skipping from one topic to an unrelated topic. (PSY)

▶ A client who has conversion disorder may display *la belle indifférence,* a lack of concern about an overwhelming disorder, such as blindness or paralysis. (PSY)

▶ *Valsalva's maneuver* is forced exhalation against a closed glottis. Cardiac patients should avoid it. (M-S)

▶ Administering chlorpromazine (Thorazine) to a client with alcohol intoxication may lead to oversedation and respiratory depression. (M-S)

▶ Vital organ perfusion is seriously compromised when mean arterial pressure decreases to less than 60 mm Hg and systolic blood pressure decreases to less than 80 mm Hg.   (M-S)

▶ Lidocaine (Xylocaine) is the drug of choice to treat premature ventricular contractions.   (M-S)

▶ The ventricles usually sustain the greatest damage during a myocardial infarction.   (M-S)

▶ During a myocardial infarction, pain occurs when anoxia causes myocardial ischemia.   (M-S)

▶ The leading cause of death in burn victims is respiratory compromise. (M-S)

▶ Overproduction of prolactin by the pituitary gland can cause galactorrhea and amenorrhea.   (M-S)

▶ When using Clark's rule, the nurse multiplies the adult dosage by the child's weight in pounds and then divides the result by 150.   (PED)

▶ When using Young's rule, the nurse multiplies the adult dosage by the child's age in years and then divides the result by the sum of the child's age plus 12.
                                                                                        (PED)

▶ A *laceration* is a torn, jagged, or irregular wound.   (FND)

▶ Wristdrop is caused by paralysis of the extensor muscles in the forearm and hand.   (M-S)

▶ Footdrop is caused by excessive plantar flexion; usually, it's a complication of prolonged bed rest.   (M-S)

▶ *Floating* occurs when the fetal presenting part isn't engaged in the pelvic inlet but is freely movable above the inlet.   (MAT)

▶ *Engagement* occurs when the largest diameter of the fetal presenting part passes through the pelvic inlet.   (MAT)

▶ In a Z-track injection, the needle track is sealed off after the injection to minimize skin irritation and staining.   (FND)

▶ The fetal station designates the relationship of the fetal presenting part to the maternal ischial spines. The number indicates the number of centimeters that the presenting part is located above or below the spines.   (MAT)

▶ A presenting part that's located above the ischial spines is designated as fetal station –1, –2, –3, or –4; a presenting part that's located below the ischial spines is designated as fetal station +1, +2, +3, or +4.   (MAT)

▶ At fetal station 0, the largest diameter of the presenting part is level with the ischial spines.   (MAT)

▶ The nurse should assess the neonate for the Moro reflex.   (MAT)

▶ *Echolalia* is the pathological parrotlike repetition of another person's words or phrases. **(PSY)**

▶ The *ego* is the rational element of the personality that maintains conscious contact with reality. **(PSY)**

▶ The *superego* is the partly conscious portion of the psyche that represents internalization of parental conscience and societal rules. It evaluates thoughts and actions, rewarding the good and punishing the bad. **(PSY)**

▶ The *id* is the unconscious part of the psyche that serves as the source of instinctual energy, impulses, and drives. **(PSY)**

▶ Ovulation ceases during pregnancy. **(MAT)**

▶ Vaginal bleeding is the most significant danger sign during pregnancy. **(MAT)**

▶ In the client who can't void, the nurse should assess the bladder first by palpation. **(M-S)**

▶ Infants younger than age 1 shouldn't receive cow's milk because of its low linoleic acid and protein content. **(PED)**

▶ A client who uses a cane should carry it on the unaffected side. **(FND)**

▶ The nurse should advise pregnant clients that no amount of alcohol intake is safe during pregnancy. **(MAT)**

▶ Vitamin C deficiency causes brittle bones, pinpoint peripheral hemorrhages, and friable gums with loose teeth. **(M-S)**

▶ Seclusion is used in psychiatric settings to ensure the client's safety. **(PSY)**

▶ *Validation* is a communication process in which the nurse confirms that she has understood the client. **(FND)**

▶ Leukemia is the most common form of cancer in children. **(M-S)**

▶ *Variability* is any change in the fetal heart rate from the normal rate of 120 to 160 beats/minute. **(MAT)**

▶ Hexachlorophene (pHisoHex) is no longer used to bathe infants because it may cause neurotoxicity. **(PED)**

▶ Rapid onset of high fever is a classic first sign of toxic shock syndrome. **(M-S)**

▶ The nurse should provide a dark, quiet environment for the neonate who's experiencing withdrawal from opioids. **(PED)**

▶ To assess jaundice in the neonate, the nurse applies slight pressure to cause blanching of the tip of the nose or the gum line, releases the pressure, and then watches for yellow discoloration. **(MAT)**

▶ In a child, the normal fasting blood glucose level is 60 to 100 mg/dl. **(PED)**

▶ If the body can't use glucose for energy production, it metabolizes fat for energy. This process results in the production of ketones. **(M-S)**

▶ Nostril flaring and inspiratory grunting are the first signs of respiratory distress in the premature neonate. **(MAT)**

▶ The infant's first emotional response is the need for affection. **(PED)**

▶ Having an imaginary friend and speaking to this friend are normal behaviors in a 3-year-old child. **(PED)**

▶ The first immunizations that a child should receive are hepatitis vaccine, diphtheria and tetanus toxoids and pertussis vaccine, and polio vaccine. **(PED)**

▶ An infant who has had diarrhea six to eight times daily for 4 consecutive days should be assessed for electrolyte imbalances. **(PED)**

▶ Cough medicines that contain codeine help suppress the cough reflex. **(FND)**

▶ Aminophylline and theophylline are bronchodilators. **(M-S)**

▶ Chest percussion helps loosen bronchial secretions. **(FND)**

▶ Skinfold measurements are used to evaluate the client's subcutaneous fat stores. **(FND)**

▶ Medulloblastomas typically occur in the cerebellum. **(M-S)**

▶ The client with diabetic ketoacidosis is at risk for shock. **(M-S)**

▶ The client with diabetes mellitus is susceptible to atherosclerosis. **(M-S)**

▶ Instilling phenylephrine (Neo-Synephrine) into the client's eye should cause mydriasis. **(M-S)**

▶ When assessing distance vision, the nurse should have the client stand 20′ (6.1 m) from the vision chart. **(FND)**

▶ An elixir, which is used mainly as a vehicle for an oral drug, contains alcohol, sweeteners, or flavorings. **(M-S)**

▶ The *basal metabolic rate* is the amount of energy needed to maintain vital body functions. **(M-S)**

▶ The basal metabolic rate is expressed in calories consumed per hour per kilogram of body weight. **(M-S)**

▶ Tetany may result from hypocalcemia. **(M-S)**

▶ Alcohol interferes with the absorption of vitamin B_{12} in the GI tract. **(M-S)**

▶ *Proteins* are the major sources of building material for muscles, blood, skin, hair, nails, and internal organs. **(FND)**

▶ A client who's taking clomipramine (Anafranil) for depression should use a sunblock to prevent a photosensitivity reaction.   (M-S)

▶ Red blood cells transport hemoglobin, white blood cells fight infection, and platelets promote coagulation.   (FND)

▶ A *compulsion* is an irresistible urge to perform an irrational act, such as walking in a clockwise circle before leaving a room or repeatedly washing one's hands.   (PSY)

▶ The therapeutic serum level for lithium is 0.6 to 1.2 mEq/L.   (PSY)

▶ *Habitual abortion* is three or more consecutive spontaneous abortions (also called *miscarriages*).   (MAT)

▶ Potassium is the most abundant cation in intracellular fluid.   (M-S)

▶ A lymph node biopsy that shows Reed-Sternberg cells provides a definitive diagnosis of Hodgkin's disease.   (M-S)

▶ The saliva of a client with rabies contains the rabies virus and thus poses a hazard to nurses who care for the client.   (M-S)

▶ A four-point (quad) cane is indicated for a client who needs more stability than a regular cane can offer.   (M-S)

▶ Excessive sedation may cause respiratory depression.   (M-S)

▶ The intraoperative period begins when the client is moved to the operating room bed and ends when he's admitted to the postanesthesia recovery unit.   (M-S)

▶ In the preoperative period, the nurse's primary concern is maintaining a patent airway.   (M-S)

▶ Cyanosis in the circumoral area, the sublingual region, or the nail beds signals oxygen saturation of less than 80%.   (M-S)

▶ During the postoperative period, the nurse should instruct the client to cough and breathe deeply every 2 hours.   (M-S)

▶ During the client's first postoperative ambulation, the nurse should keep a close watch and assist as needed.   (M-S)

▶ Hypovolemia occurs when 15% to 25% of the body's total blood volume is lost.   (M-S)

▶ In postoperative clients, the organism that's most likely to cause septicemia is *Escherichia coli*.   (M-S)

▶ Teenage mothers are at increased risk for having low-birth-weight neonates.   (MAT)

▶ Before drawing blood to measure arterial blood gases, the nurse should perform Allen's test to check the client's collateral blood supply.   (M-S)

▶ A drug has three names: a generic name; a trade, or brand, name; and a chemical name. **(FND)**

▶ The nurse should keep suction equipment at the bedside of the client who's recovering from maxillofacial surgery. **(M-S)**

▶ *Bestiality* is sexual relations between a human being and an animal. **(PSY)**

▶ *Crowning* is the appearance of the fetus's head as it becomes visible at the vulvovaginal ring and its largest diameter is encircled. **(MAT)**

▶ If an immunization schedule is interrupted, it should resume from the last immunization administered, not from the beginning. **(PED)**

▶ *Passive exercises* are performed by one person on another. **(FND)**

▶ *Resistance exercises* are performed by one person against the resistance of another. **(FND)**

▶ In *isometric exercises*, the person contracts his muscles without moving the affected body part. **(FND)**

▶ Activities of daily living are the activities that a person performs during the course of a normal day. **(FND)**

▶ Cardiopulmonary resuscitation shouldn't be interrupted unless the rescuer is alone and must stop to get help. **(M-S)**

▶ The tongue is the most common cause of airway obstruction in unconscious clients. **(M-S)**

▶ If a client has an amputation, advise against using lotion or powder on the stump. **(M-S)**

▶ In balloon angioplasty, a small, balloon-tipped catheter is inflated inside an artery to exert pressure against a plaque and flatten it. **(M-S)**

▶ The client who has a stomach ulcer should avoid bedtime snacks because food may stimulate nocturnal gastric secretions. **(M-S)**

▶ A clear liquid diet consists of clear fluids and foods that become liquid at body temperature. **(FND)**

▶ A full liquid diet consists of simple, easily digested foods. This diet provides fluids and calories but may be inadequate in folic acid, iron, vitamin B_6, and fiber. **(FND)**

▶ A pureed diet supplies all of the client's nutritional needs. **(M-S)**

▶ A soft diet includes semisolid foods and is typically supplemented with between-meal snacks. **(FND)**

▶ A mechanical soft diet is used for the client who has difficulty chewing or tolerating a regular diet. **(FND)**

▶ The client who requires no dietary modifications can receive a regular diet.
(FND)

▶ The physician normally orders a "diet for age" for the pediatric client. (PED)

▶ A bland diet doesn't include foods that cause gastric irritation or excess acid secretions unless they provide a neutralizing effect. (FND)

▶ The client who has a gastric ulcer should avoid alcohol, caffeinated beverages, aspirin, and spicy foods. (M-S)

▶ Bacteria that convert penicillin into an inactive product produce the enzyme penicillinase. (M-S)

▶ Staphylococcal or streptococcal organisms cause impetigo contagiosa. (M-S)

▶ *Battle's sign* is bluish discoloration or bruising over the mastoid area and indicates a basal skull fracture. (M-S)

▶ Antibiotics are ineffective against viruses, protozoa, and parasites. (M-S)

▶ Natural penicillins inhibit synthesis of the bacterial cell wall. (M-S)

▶ Aminoglycosides are natural antibiotics that are effective against gram-negative bacteria. (M-S)

▶ When caring for a client who's receiving aminoglycosides, the nurse should watch for nephrotoxicity and ototoxicity. (M-S)

▶ In *phimosis,* the foreskin can't be retracted over the glans penis. (PED)

▶ A client with a strangulated hernia typically has pain, nausea, and vomiting.
(M-S)

▶ In chronic prostatitis, the prostate gland is enlarged, tender, and somewhat boggy. (M-S)

▶ At age 5 to 6 months, an infant can tell one face from another and will exhibit stranger anxiety. (PED)

▶ To perform the cardinal positions of gaze, the nurse asks the client to remain still while she holds a pencil or other small object directly in front of his nose at a distance of 18" (45.7 cm). Then she asks him to follow the object with his eyes without moving his head. (M-S)

▶ The six cardinal positions of gaze evaluate the oculomotor, trigeminal, and abducent nerves as well as the extraocular muscles. (M-S)

▶ Abnormal findings when performing the cardinal movements of gaze include nystagmus and amblyopia. (M-S)

▶ The six cardinal movements of gaze are right superior, right lateral, left superior, left lateral, right inferior, and left inferior. (M-S)

▶ A *hordeolum* (stye) is an inflammation of the eyelid margin that originates in a sebaceous gland of an eyelash. **(M-S)**

▶ A *chalazion* is chronic eyelid inflammation that's caused by an obstructed meibomian gland. **(M-S)**

▶ Respiratory acidosis may occur in such conditions as drug overdose, Guillain-Barré syndrome, myasthenia gravis, and chronic obstructive pulmonary disease. **(M-S)**

▶ Respiratory alkalosis may occur in such conditions as high fever, severe hypoxia, asthma, and pulmonary embolism. **(M-S)**

▶ Metabolic acidosis may result from renal failure, diarrhea, diabetic ketosis, or lactic ketosis. **(M-S)**

▶ Metabolic alkalosis may result from nasal and gastric suctioning, excessive diuretic use, or steroid therapy. **(M-S)**

▶ Heart murmurs occur in six grades, designated I through VI. **(M-S)**

▶ The nurse can hear a grade VI heart murmur with the stethoscope raised slightly above the client's chest. **(M-S)**

▶ The "six Fs" of abdominal distention are flatus, feces, fetus, fluid, fat, and fatal growth neoplasm. **(FND)**

▶ Murphy's sign indicates acute cholecystitis. **(M-S)**

▶ *Psoas sign* (abdominal rigidity and rebound tenderness) indicates appendicitis. **(M-S)**

▶ The nurse can detect ascites by checking for a fluid wave in the abdomen or by percussing the abdomen for shifting dullness. **(FND)**

▶ The client's goal is the most important goal to incorporate into the nursing care plan. **(FND)**

▶ A stable environment helps minimize confusion in the client with organic brain syndrome. **(PSY)**

▶ Typically, the client with organic brain syndrome loses recent memory first. **(PSY)**

▶ The *Apgar score* indicates the neonate's respiratory effort, heart rate, muscle tone, reflex irritability, and color. It's obtained 1 and 5 minutes after birth. **(MAT)**

▶ During cardiac catheterization, the client may experience a thudding sensation in the chest as a result of manipulating the catheter. **(M-S)**

▶ During the third trimester of pregnancy, the anti-insulin effects of placental hormones increase the client's insulin needs. **(MAT)**

▶ During ultrasound, the biparietal diameter of the fetal head is used to assess gestational age. **(MAT)**

▶ Congenital malformations are common in neonates of diabetic mothers. **(MAT)**

▶ Nutritional deficiency is a common finding in clients with a long-standing history of alcohol abuse. **(PSY)**

▶ An alcoholic client typically receives thiamine to slow the progression of peripheral neuropathy. **(PSY)**

▶ A client who's experiencing alcohol withdrawal may receive sedatives to prevent delirium tremens. **(PSY)**

▶ Alcohol lowers the seizure threshold in some people. **(PSY)**

▶ *Paraphrasing* is an active listening technique in which the nurse restates the message that the client has just conveyed. **(FND)**

▶ During the *preicteric phase* of hepatitis A infection, early signs and symptoms include headache, malaise, fatigue, lassitude, anorexia, and fever. **(M-S)**

▶ Most clients with hepatitis A infection are asymptomatic. **(M-S)**

▶ Hepatitis A usually spreads by the fecal-oral route. **(M-S)**

▶ A significant increase in the serum transaminase level is characteristic of both hepatitis A and hepatitis B. **(M-S)**

▶ Excessive vomiting or suctioning of the stomach contents can reduce body stores of potassium and cause hypokalemia. **(M-S)**

▶ Signs of acute rheumatic fever include chorea, fever, carditis, migratory polyarthritis, skin rash, and subcutaneous nodules. **(M-S)**

▶ A client who has a history of rheumatic fever should take prophylactic antibiotics before undergoing dental work or other invasive procedures. **(M-S)**

▶ A client who's following a low-residue diet should avoid fruit because it's high in fiber and low in protein. **(M-S)**

▶ Postoperative pain peaks during the first 24 hours after surgery. **(M-S)**

▶ After a myocardial infarction, most clients are permitted to resume sexual activity when they can climb two flights of stairs without fatigue or dyspnea. **(M-S)**

▶ Geriatric clients are more susceptible to orthostatic hypotension than younger clients. **(M-S)**

▶ Tightening the buttocks is a perineal exercise that strengthens the pelvic muscles. **(M-S)**

▶ When two psychiatric clients are engaged in escalating hostilities, the nurse should defuse the situation by sending both clients to their rooms and providing one-on-one therapy. (PSY)

▶ Many preterm neonates have immature swallowing and sucking reflexes. (MAT)

▶ The nurse should strain the urine of the client who has suspected renal or urethral calculi to determine whether any calculi have passed. (M-S)

▶ The nurse should inventory and safeguard the personal belongings of the deceased adult client. (FND)

▶ To maximize lung expansion, the nurse should place the client with ascites in the semi-Fowler position. (M-S)

▶ When caring for the client who has ingested poison, the nurse should save vomitus for analysis. (M-S)

▶ Acrocyanosis and cool extremities are normal findings in neonates. (MAT)

▶ The earliest signs of respiratory distress are restlessness and an increased respiratory rate, followed by an increased heart rate. (M-S)

▶ Vomiting within 4 hours after a meal may be caused by food intoxication as a result of bacterial toxins. (M-S)

▶ Vomiting, fever, and diarrhea that occur 12 to 18 hours after a meal suggest food poisoning. (M-S)

▶ The client who's receiving loop diuretics should supplement his diet with foods that contain potassium. (M-S)

▶ For the confused client, maintaining consistency in nursing staff is important. (PSY)

▶ *Hypercapnia* is an excess of carbon dioxide in the blood. (M-S)

▶ Vasopressin and oxytocin are secreted by the posterior pituitary gland. (M-S)

▶ Signs and symptoms of hypothyroidism include dry, coarse, flaky skin and hair; a thick tongue; and cold intolerance. (M-S)

▶ For a client with hypothyroidism, administer one-third to one-half the normal dose of sedatives, as ordered, to reduce the risk of oversedation. (M-S)

▶ A client with hyperthyroidism should avoid stimulants found in some drugs and foods. (M-S)

▶ Before an eye examination with an ophthalmoscope, have the client remove his contact lenses (if they are tinted) or remove his eyeglasses. (FND)

▶ When using crutches, the client should bear weight on the hands. (FND)

▶ The female reproductive organs that are normally affected by gonorrhea are the vagina and fallopian tubes. (M-S)

▶ After surgery to correct retinal detachment, the client should avoid sudden movement, such as sneezing or bending over. (M-S)

▶ Hemorrhage is the most common postoperative problem. (M-S)

▶ *Kussmaul's respirations* are the body's attempt to "blow off" excess carbon dioxide. (M-S)

▶ *Phenylketonuria* is an inborn error of metabolism of phenylalanine. (PED)

▶ *Epinephrine hydrochloride* is a sympathomimetic drug that acts primarily on alpha$_1$, beta$_1$, and beta$_2$ receptors. (M-S)

▶ Adverse effects of epinephrine hydrochloride administration include tachycardia, palpitations, headache, and hypertension. (M-S)

▶ Signs and symptoms of cystitis include frequency of urination, lower abdominal discomfort, dysuria, and dribbling. (M-S)

▶ The nurse should use mild soap and water to clean the skin around a stoma. (M-S)

▶ Green, leafy vegetables are high in fiber. (FND)

▶ A cardinal sign of acute pancreatitis is an elevated serum amylase level. (M-S)

▶ During colostomy irrigation, painful cramps may result from a rapid flow rate. (M-S)

▶ The client can control some of the odor associated with a colostomy by avoiding such foods as fish, eggs, onions, beans, and cabbage. (M-S)

▶ The average child requires a 25G to 27G ½" needle for subcutaneous injections. (PED)

▶ When injecting less than 1 ml of a drug subcutaneously, the nurse should use a tuberculin syringe. (FND)

▶ Before administering medication, the nurse must identify the client by checking his identification band. (FND)

▶ Before giving an injection, the nurse should clean the skin at the injection site with a sterile alcohol pad, starting at the center and moving outward in circles. (FND)

▶ If blood is aspirated into the syringe before an I.M. injection, the nurse should withdraw the needle without injecting the medication and should prepare another syringe. (FND)

▶ After an injection, the nurse should apply pressure to the injection site to stop bleeding. (FND)

▶ The nurse should never tweeze a client's eyebrows or dye a client's hair.
(FND)

▶ When providing hair and scalp care, the nurse should start combing at the ends of the hair and work toward the scalp. (FND)

▶ The nurse shouldn't cut the client's hair without written consent from the client, parent, or guardian. (FND)

▶ When washing her hands, the nurse need not remove a wedding ring but should remove a watch and other jewelry. (FND)

▶ When caring for a hearing-impaired client, the nurse should raise her voice moderately but shouldn't shout. (FND)

▶ Redness after the application of a heat lamp indicates a skin burn. (M-S)

▶ The nurse should remove the client's heel protectors every 8 hours to expose the heels to air and to assess the skin. (M-S)

▶ Hot soaks promote drainage and relieve pain from inflammation. (FND)

▶ The most common sexually transmitted disease in the United States is chlamydia (M-S)

▶ In women, signs of chlamydial infection include a positive culture, urinary frequency, greenish white vaginal discharge, and cervical inflammation.
(M-S)

▶ The pituitary gland is located in the sella turcica of the sphenoid bone in the cranial cavity. (M-S)

▶ Healing by secondary intention occurs with large wounds that cause significant tissue loss. (M-S)

▶ In healing by first intention, union or continuity occurs directly and the wound edges are well approximated, usually with sutures. (M-S)

▶ Myasthenia gravis typically affects young women. (M-S)

▶ Clients with anorexia nervosa must be observed during meals and for several hours afterward. (PSY)

▶ A child with untreated phenylketonuria doesn't reach early developmental milestones. (PED)

▶ Degenerative joint disease is the most common form of arthritis that affects almost all joints. (M-S)

▶ Osteoarthritis causes progressive deterioration and loss of articular cartilage.
(M-S)

▶ Reactive arthritis typically causes conjunctivitis and urethritis as well as arthritis. (M-S)

▶ Foods that are high in carbohydrates are quickly digested, are readily emptied from the stomach into the duodenum, and are likely to cause diarrhea. **(M-S)**

▶ Drying the neonate immediately after delivery helps maintain body heat by preventing heat loss through evaporation. **(MAT)**

▶ When bathing an infant, the nurse should expose only one body part at a time. **(MAT)**

▶ To promote bonding, the mother should be permitted to breast-feed her neonate on the delivery table. **(MAT)**

▶ The nurse should measure the neonate's temperature at least every 2 hours. **(MAT)**

▶ Typically, a neonate weighs 5.5 to 9 lb (2.5 to 4 kg) and measures 18" to 22" (45.5 to 56 cm) long. **(MAT)**

▶ To test the patency of the nares, the nurse should try to elicit a sneeze from the neonate. **(MAT)**

▶ *Epstein's pearls* (pseudodiphtheria) are small, whitish yellow lesions that may appear on either side of the neonate's throat. They are normal and disappear without treatment. **(MAT)**

▶ Supernumerary nipples occasionally appear on neonates and may be mistaken for moles. **(MAT)**

▶ Signs and symptoms of chronic renal failure include decreased urine output, Kussmaul's respirations, and uremic frost. **(M-S)**

▶ *Polydactyly* is extra fingers or toes. **(M-S)**

▶ Babinski's reflex is normal in the neonate and may persist for as long as 18 months. **(MAT)**

▶ In the *extrusion reflex*, the infant spits out food that's placed on the front of the tongue. **(PED)**

▶ *Harlequin sign* is reddening of the lower half of the body and pallor of the upper half in the neonate who's lying on his side. **(MAT)**

▶ *Mongolian spots* are blue-black macules that are seen on the sacrum and buttocks of some neonates. **(MAT)**

▶ *Vernix caseosa* is a cheeselike substance that covers the skin of the neonate. **(MAT)**

▶ A *fugue state* is an extreme form of amnesia that's accompanied by flight from familiar surroundings; the person may take on a new identity. **(PSY)**

▶ When administering penicillin G procaine I.M. to the adult, the nurse should inject the needle deep into the upper outer quadrant of the buttock. **(M-S)**

▶ *Caput succedaneum* in the fetus is scalp swelling that may overlie the sutures of the skull. Usually, it occurs during labor as a result of pressure exerted by the cervix. **(MAT)**

▶ *Nevus flammeus* (port-wine stain) is a diffuse lesion that ranges from pink to dark bluish red and may appear on the neonate's face or thighs. **(MAT)**

▶ *Strawberry hemangiomas* are raised, red birthmarks that usually disappear by age 1 year. **(MAT)**

▶ *Cavernous hemangiomas* resemble strawberry hemangiomas but don't disappear with age. **(M-S)**

▶ For the neonate's first bottle-feeding, the nurse should give him a few sips of sterile water followed by 1 oz of glucose water. **(MAT)**

▶ To help establish the mother's milk supply pattern, the breast-fed neonate should be fed at least every 2 to 3 hours. **(MAT)**

▶ The neonate who has a suspected infection should be isolated. **(PED)**

▶ The Schilling test confirms the diagnosis of pernicious anemia. **(M-S)**

▶ A colostomy in the ascending colon drains fluid fecal matter. **(M-S)**

▶ A colostomy in the descending colon drains solid fecal matter. **(M-S)**

▶ A client who's undergoing chemotherapy should eat a diet that's high in calories and protein. **(M-S)**

▶ Chemotherapy may cause hair loss. Clients who need chemotherapy should be told to expect this effect. **(M-S)**

▶ The infant with celiac disease has fatty, foul-smelling feces. **(PED)**

▶ The results of hemoglobin electrophoresis differentiate sickle cell trait from sickle cell anemia. **(M-S)**

▶ *Eruption* is the emergence of a tooth from the dental crypt and through the surrounding tissue. **(PED)**

▶ A folded towel (scrotal bridge) can be used to provide scrotal support after scrotal surgery. **(M-S)**

▶ In a pregnant woman, supine hypotension syndrome occurs when the enlarging uterus exerts pressure that decreases venous return. **(MAT)**

▶ The nurse should advise the pregnant client who has ankle edema to rest frequently, elevate her feet, and avoid constrictive clothing. **(MAT)**

▶ When a physician orders "diet as tolerated," the nurse should progress the client's diet as follows: clear liquids, full liquids, soft diet, and regular (house) diet. **(M-S)**

▶ Drinking too much plain water can lead to electrolyte imbalances. **(FND)**

▶ The client has the right to accept or refuse treatment.   **(FND)**

▶ Illness or injury may cause a person to regress to a lower level of functioning.   **(FND)**

▶ *Health* is a state of physiologic and psychological well-being.   **(FND)**

▶ In naturally acquired active immunity, antibodies are produced after exposure to a microorganism.   **(M-S)**

▶ Naturally acquired passive immunity occurs when the fetus receives antibodies from the mother.   **(MAT)**

▶ In artificially acquired immunity, a person is infected with weakened or dead microorganisms or with an inactive form of the organism's toxin.   **(M-S)**

▶ The major types of tissue are epithelial, connective, muscle, and nerve.   **(M-S)**

▶ Cells are the body's basic structural unit.   **(FND)**

▶ During the aging process, bones lose calcium and become brittle. This change increases the risk of fractures and poor healing after a fracture.   **(FND)**

▶ Because damage to dermal skin causes loss of the skin's mitotic structures, the damaged dermis takes longer to heal than the damaged epidermis.   **(M-S)**

▶ Diffusion, osmosis, and filtration are passive transport processes.   **(M-S)**

▶ The main types of muscle tissue are skeletal (voluntary), smooth (involuntary), and cardiac.   **(M-S)**

▶ Neurons respond to stimuli and transmit nerve impulses.   **(M-S)**

▶ Neuroglia support and connect nervous tissue but don't transmit nerve impulses.   **(M-S)**

▶ Multiple sclerosis causes deterioration of the myelin sheath of the central nervous system. (Think "MS" for multiple sclerosis and myelin sheath.)   **(M-S)**

▶ The body has 31 pairs of spinal nerves.   **(M-S)**

▶ The thyroid gland controls the rate of metabolism.   **(M-S)**

▶ The parathyroid gland regulates serum calcium and phosphorus levels. **(M-S)**

▶ Blood is composed of plasma and formed elements (white blood cells, red blood cells, and platelets).   **(M-S)**

▶ A client who's on nothing-by-mouth (NPO) status for 3 days or longer without receiving nutritional support is at risk for nutritional deficits.   **(M-S)**

▶ If a client has nausea or starts to choke or vomit during a tube feeding, the nurse should stop the feeding immediately and call the physician.   **(M-S)**

▶ The nurse should check the client's distal pulses before and after splinting a fracture.   **(M-S)**

▶ Rescuers who are performing cardiopulmonary resuscitation on a child should deliver 100 chest compressions per minute. **(PED)**

▶ A client who has a completely obstructed airway can't talk, breathe, or cough. **(M-S)**

▶ The courts are likely to assume that nursing care that wasn't documented wasn't performed. **(FND)**

▶ During skin allergy testing, the nurse should keep epinephrine and emergency equipment available. **(M-S)**

▶ Alcohol is a central nervous system depressant. **(M-S)**

▶ Gangrene usually affects the fingers and toes first. **(M-S)**

▶ In the infant, a sunken fontanel is one of the first signs of dehydration. Others include decreased tearing and decreased urine output. **(PED)**

▶ A trauma victim shouldn't be moved until a patent airway is established and the cervical spine is immobilized. **(M-S)**

▶ Rescuers should place the victim on a solid, flat surface before administering cardiopulmonary resuscitation. **(M-S)**

▶ Brain damage occurs 4 to 6 minutes after cardiopulmonary function ceases. **(M-S)**

▶ An adrenalectomy may decrease steroid production and lead to extensive sodium and water loss. **(M-S)**

▶ In a healthy person, fluid intake roughly equals fluid loss. **(M-S)**

▶ The body's major buffer system is the bicarbonate buffer. **(M-S)**

▶ Metabolic acidosis results from excessive loss of bicarbonate or excessive production or retention of acid. **(M-S)**

▶ *Hemianopia* is blindness or defective vision in one-half of the visual field of one or both eyes. **(FND)**

▶ After a fracture of the epiphyseal plate, the child may have growth disturbances, such as bone shortening or overgrowth. **(PED)**

▶ An acetaminophen overdose can severely damage the liver and can lead to liver failure or death. **(M-S)**

▶ Prominent signs of advanced cirrhosis are ascites and jaundice. **(M-S)**

▶ *Somnambulism* is sleepwalking. **(M-S)**

▶ Epinephrine is a vasoconstrictor. **(M-S)**

▶ Stress management is a short-term goal of psychotherapy. **(PSY)**

▶ Penicillin should be administered 1 to 2 hours before or 2 to 3 hours after a meal. (M-S)

▶ To ensure accurate central venous pressure readings, the nurse should place the manometer or transducer level with the phlebostatic axis. (M-S)

▶ Arterial blood is bright red, flows rapidly, and spurts with each heartbeat because it's pumped directly from the heart. (M-S)

▶ Venous blood is dark red and tends to ooze from a wound. (M-S)

▶ Signs and symptoms of anaphylaxis commonly stem from histamine release. (M-S)

▶ Urine pH of greater than 8.0 can result from a urinary tract infection, a highly alkaline diet, or systemic alkalosis. (M-S)

▶ Urine pH of less than 4.5 may indicate a high-protein diet, fever, or metabolic acidosis. (M-S)

▶ Signs of accessory muscle use include elevation of the shoulder, retraction of the intercostal muscles, and use of the scalene and sternocleidomastoid muscles during respiration. (M-S)

▶ *Lanugo* is the fine, downy hair that covers the fetus's body. It's almost entirely shed by 40 weeks' gestation. (MAT)

▶ If wound dehiscence occurs, the nurse should cover the wound with a moist, sterile dressing and notify the physician. The protruding intestine should be moistened continually and not allowed to dry out. (M-S)

▶ A rash is the most common allergic reaction to penicillin. (M-S)

▶ Atropine blocks the effects of acetylcholine. (M-S)

▶ Patent ductus arteriosus is an acyanotic congenital heart defect. (M-S)

▶ Salicylates are the drugs of choice to treat rheumatoid arthritis. (M-S)

▶ Deep, intense pain that worsens at night and is unrelated to movement suggests bone pain. (M-S)

▶ Pain that occurs after prolonged or excessive exercise and subsides with rest suggests muscle pain. (M-S)

▶ Mannitol (Osmitrol) is an osmotic diuretic. (M-S)

▶ The *biophysical profile* is a scoring system used to assess fetal well-being. (MAT)

▶ TORCH infections include toxoplasmosis, other infections (chlamydia, group B beta-hemolytic streptococcus, syphilis, and varicella zoster), rubella, cytomegalovirus, and herpesviruses. (M-S)

▶ Red cell indices aid in diagnosing anemias. (M-S)

▶ Before transferring the client from a bed to a wheelchair, the nurse should push the wheelchair's footrests to the sides and lock the wheels.   **(FND)**

▶ Tetralogy of Fallot consists of four defects: ventricular septal defect, overriding aorta, pulmonic stenosis, and right ventricular hypertrophy.   **(PED)**

▶ An exercise stress test is continued until the client reaches a predetermined target heart rate or has chest pain, fatigue, or other signs or symptoms of exercise intolerance.   **(M-S)**

▶ The therapeutic blood level for digoxin is 0.5 to 2.5 ng/ml.   **(M-S)**

▶ Under the Controlled Substances Act, the pharmacy must account for every dose of a controlled drug that it dispenses.   **(FND)**

▶ Jaundice is a sign of dysfunction, not a disease in itself.   **(M-S)**

▶ Most clients who have type 2 diabetes mellitus don't need exogenous insulin.   **(M-S)**

▶ Intermediate-acting insulin levels peak in 4 to 15 hours.   **(M-S)**

▶ Long-acting insulin levels peak in 10 to 30 hours.   **(M-S)**

▶ Hypoglycemia occurs when the blood glucose level is less than 50 mg/dl.   **(M-S)**

▶ Hypoglycemia may occur 1 to 3 hours after the administration of a rapid-acting insulin.   **(M-S)**

▶ A rapid decrease in the blood glucose level may cause sweating, tremors, pallor, and tachycardia.   **(M-S)**

▶ A person who has diabetes mellitus should inspect his feet daily for corns and blisters.   **(M-S)**

▶ Corrective lenses for nearsightedness are concave.   **(M-S)**

▶ Corrective lenses for farsightedness are convex.   **(M-S)**

▶ *Refraction* is the clinical measurement of refractive errors of the eye.   **(FND)**

▶ *Adhesions* are bands of granulation and scar tissue that develop in some clients after a surgical incision.   **(M-S)**

▶ The nurse should moisten an eye patch when applying it on an unconscious client, making sure the client's eye is closed.   **(FND)**

▶ The fluorescent treponemal antibody absorption test is a specific serologic test for syphilis.   **(M-S)**

▶ Signs of circulatory interference include abnormally cool skin, cyanosis, and rubor or pallor.   **(M-S)**

▶ The Hoyer lift allows two people to lift and move a nonambulatory client safely.   **(FND)**

▶ The nurse should use a vest restraint cautiously in a client who has heart failure. The restraint may tighten with movement, further limiting respiratory function. **(FND)**

▶ The Centers for Disease Control and Prevention recommends using a needleless system when piggybacking an I.V. medication into the main I.V. line. **(M-S)**

▶ A mask should cover the wearer's mouth and nose. It shouldn't be used longer than 30 minutes or be reused. **(FND)**

▶ If a gown is required, the nurse should put it on before entering the client's room and discard it on leaving. **(FND)**

▶ The average duration of a pregnancy is 280 days, 40 weeks, 9 calendar months, or 10 lunar months. **(MAT)**

▶ The nurse should suspect respiratory alkalosis in a client whose partial pressure of carbon dioxide is less than 35 mm Hg. **(M-S)**

▶ A *vitamin* is an organic compound that's essential to metabolic processes and can't be synthesized by the body. **(M-S)**

▶ The peer group is a major influence on the adolescent's eating habits. **(PED)**

▶ Respiratory tract infections may trigger asthma attacks. **(M-S)**

▶ Oxygen therapy is used to prevent or treat hypoxemia in the client with severe asthma. **(M-S)**

▶ During an asthma attack, the client may prefer nasal prongs to a Venturi mask because the mask may have a smothering effect. **(M-S)**

▶ Cellulitis causes localized heat, redness, swelling and, occasionally, fever, chills, and malaise. **(M-S)**

▶ The neonate's hemoglobin value is normally 14 to 27 g/dl. **(MAT)**

▶ Venous stasis may trigger thrombophlebitis. **(M-S)**

▶ *Vitiligo* is a skin disease caused by the destruction of pigment cells. It causes irregular skin patches that lack pigment. **(M-S)**

▶ Ascites may be detected when more than 500 ml of fluid has accumulated in the intraperitoneal space. **(M-S)**

▶ In adults, gastroenteritis is usually self-limiting and causes diarrhea, abdominal discomfort, nausea, and vomiting. **(M-S)**

▶ A client who's recovering from surgery to correct retinal detachment should avoid sudden movements because they put stress on the suture line. **(M-S)**

▶ Taut, shiny skin and edema are signs of excess fluid volume. **(M-S)**

▶ On percussion, dullness is heard over the liver. **(FND)**

▶ When a client has suspected food poisoning after eating at a restaurant, the nurse should notify public health authorities, who will take samples of the suspected contaminated food and interview the client, food handlers, and other patrons of the restaurant. (M-S)

▶ Down syndrome (trisomy 21) is the most common chromosomal disorder. (PED)

▶ When determining how to explain a procedure to a hospitalized child, the nurse should consider the child's developmental age. (PED)

▶ Angiotensin-converting enzyme inhibitors decrease blood pressure by interfering with the renin-angiotensin-aldosterone system. (M-S)

▶ An *anion* is an ion that carries a negative electrical charge. (M-S)

▶ *Urinary incontinence* is the inability to voluntarily control urination. (M-S)

▶ Clients who have a spinal cord injury at or above T7 are at risk for autonomic dysreflexia. (M-S)

▶ *Bradypnea* is a respiratory rate of fewer than 12 breaths/minute. (FND)

▶ *Residual volume* is the amount of air that remains in the lungs after the deepest possible expiration. (FND)

▶ Nitrofurantoin (Macrodantin) may turn the urine brown or darker in color. (M-S)

▶ In a dark-skinned client, jaundice may not be observable in the sclera. (FND)

▶ Handling a wet cast with the fingertips instead of the palms of the hands can cause indentations in the cast that may lead to pressure ulcers. (FND)

▶ Informed consent is required for any invasive procedure. (FND)

▶ A phenytoin level of 10 to 20 mcg/ml is therapeutic. (M-S)

▶ In an infant, a key sign of increasing intracranial pressure is a bulging fontanelle. (PED)

▶ In *phantom sensation,* the client feels as though the missing body part, such as a breast or limb, is still present. (M-S)

▶ *Dysfunctional grief* is grief that's abnormal or distorted and may be inhibited or unresolved. (PSY)

▶ The normal value for arterial blood oxygen saturation is 94% to 100%. (M-S)

▶ One milliliter is equivalent to 30 cm^3. (FND)

▶ When using crutches, bearing weight on the axillae can damage the nerves and circulation in that area. (FND)

▶ The Rh-negative woman who isn't sensitized should receive $Rh_o(D)$ immune globulin after an abortion.   (MAT)

▶ If a client is receiving propranolol (Inderal), the nurse should tell the client not to discontinue the drug suddenly because doing so could exacerbate angina.   (M-S)

▶ The radial artery is most commonly used to obtain an arterial blood gas measurement.   (M-S)

▶ The nurse should warn the client who's receiving phenytoin (Dilantin) that it may turn the urine pink, red, or reddish brown.   (M-S)

▶ Feeding patterns for the bottle-fed infant are every 3 to 4 hours on demand.   (PED)

▶ Measures to prevent transmission of infection include hand washing, barrier precautions, and isolation precautions.   (FND)

▶ A *syrup* is a drug combined with water and a sugar solution.   (FND)

▶ The enzyme-linked immunosorbent assay determines the presence of human immunodeficiency virus antibodies and documents exposure to the virus.   (M-S)

▶ The fourth stage of labor ends with maternal stabilization and lasts 1 to 2 hours.   (MAT)

▶ Almost all external bleeding can be stopped by direct pressure.   (M-S)

▶ Verapamil (Calan) is a calcium channel blocker.   (M-S)

▶ The postoperative client who's positioned upright too quickly may experience light-headedness, dizziness, and fainting.   (M-S)

▶ Raynaud's phenomenon is more common in cold climates and during the winter months.   (M-S)

▶ A disulfiram (Antabuse) reaction includes flushing, throbbing headache, dyspnea, nausea, vomiting, diaphoresis, chest pain, hyperventilation, hypotension, syncope, weakness, blurred vision, and confusion.   (M-S)

▶ Consent can be deemed legally insufficient if it can be proven that the client didn't understand all of the facts about a procedure.   (M-S)

▶ Intact skin and mucous membranes are the body's first line of defense against microorganisms.   (FND)

▶ The Western blot test identifies the presence of human immunodeficiency virus antibodies and confirms seropositivity of the enzyme-linked immunosorbent assay.   (M-S)

▶ *Desensitization therapy* gradually exposes the client to anxiety-provoking or emotionally distressing stimuli.   (PSY)

▶ One gram of carbohydrate provides 4 calories.   (M-S)

▶ Because a clear liquid diet is deficient in certain nutrients, it's suitable only for brief periods, typically 24 to 36 hours postoperatively.   (FND)

▶ When administering heparin subcutaneously, the nurse shouldn't aspirate after injection into the skin.   (M-S)

▶ The normal serum creatinine level is 0 to 200 mg/24 hours.   (M-S)

▶ If a client has gangrene of the feet, the nurse should use a bed cradle to prevent further breakdown of tissue.   (FND)

▶ A low-fat, low-sodium diet includes chicken and fresh salad.   (FND)

▶ If the client hasn't signed an informed consent form for a procedure, he shouldn't be transferred from the unit to the operating room and the charge nurse should be notified.   (FND)

▶ Iron medication should be administered after meals.   (FND)

▶ Atropine is administered preoperatively to desiccate secretions.   (M-S)

▶ Before a blood transfusion, the client is routinely given diphenhydramine hydrochloride to minimize transfusion reactions.   (M-S)

▶ A client with oral candidiasis should be instructed to keep nystatin (Mycostatin) oral solution in his mouth as long as possible to facilitate contact of the medication with the organism.   (M-S)

▶ Predisposing factors for oral cancer include smoking cigarettes, chewing tobacco, and drinking alcohol.   (M-S)

▶ The nurse should inspect the emesis of the client who has an oral cesium or radium radioactive implant to ensure that it wasn't displaced during vomiting.   (M-S)

▶ *Ecchymosis* is bruised tissue.   (M-S)

▶ *Erythema* is reddened tissue.   (M-S)

▶ To minimize and relieve edema, the nurse should elevate the client's affected limb and apply ice for 20 minutes on followed by 20 minutes off.   (M-S)

▶ When wrapping the ankle with a roller bandage, the nurse should start at the metatarsals and wrap from the distal to the proximal aspect of the foot.   (FND)

▶ Clients with varicose veins may have achiness, heaviness, and pain in the affected leg.   (M-S)

▶ *Claudication* is pain on ambulation; the most likely cause is inadequate arterial blood flow.   (M-S)

▶ The treatment for anaphylaxis is epinephrine.   (M-S)

▶ The best method to relieve the pain associated with varicose veins is to elevate the affected leg periodically throughout the day. **(M-S)**

▶ Stasis ulcers first appear as darkly pigmented, scaly areas and progress to skin breakdown and craters that are difficult to heal. **(M-S)**

▶ For the client who has had vein stripping and vein ligation surgery, the physician usually orders walking hourly in the immediate postoperative period. **(M-S)**

▶ Caffeine can impair blood flow because it constricts arteries and arterioles. It should be avoided by clients who have a history of venous stasis. **(M-S)**

▶ Signs of adequate circulation in a leg include warm toes and feet and capillary refill of less than 3 seconds. **(FND)**

▶ A throat culture is obtained from the posterior pharynx. While obtaining the culture, the nurse should avoid touching the client's tongue and mouth with the swab. **(FND)**

▶ A person who's taking antihistamines shouldn't drive or use machinery because the medication may make him drowsy. **(M-S)**

▶ An anaphylactic reaction causes dyspnea, hypotension, hives, and loss of consciousness. **(M-S)**

▶ Sequelae of untreated beta-hemolytic streptococcal infections, such as strep throat, are glomerulonephritis, rheumatic fever, and rheumatic heart disease. **(M-S)**

▶ A client who has laryngitis should rest the larynx by avoiding whispering and talking. **(M-S)**

▶ Parents should use a cool-mist humidifier rather than a steam humidifier to reduce the risk of a scalding injury to the child. **(M-S)**

▶ To minimize the risk of diversional activity deficit, the nurse should encourage the client's family and friends to visit the client and allow him to engage in enjoyable activities that are consistent with the treatment plan. **(FND)**

▶ A client who has an esophageal stricture should chew his food thoroughly; well-chewed food passes into the stomach more easily. **(M-S)**

▶ The most common symptoms of hemolytic blood transfusion reactions are dyspnea, lower back pain, constriction in the chest, and hypotension. **(M-S)**

▶ *Ineffective infant feeding pattern* is the appropriate nursing diagnosis for an infant who can't coordinate sucking, swallowing, and breathing. **(M-S)**

▶ A client who has a hiatal hernia should be instructed to sit upright for at least 2 hours after meals, sleep with his head elevated, and eat frequent small meals to avoid overextending his stomach. **(M-S)**

▶ Flank pain is a common manifestation of acute pyelonephritis. **(M-S)**

▶ The best indication of successful hyperalimentation or gastric feeding is maintenance of prehospital weight or regaining of lost weight. **(M-S)**

▶ After a gastrostomy, the nurse should expect serosanguineous draining from the gastrostomy tube. **(M-S)**

▶ *Disturbed body image* is an appropriate nursing diagnosis for a client who has bronzelike pigmentation on the face as a result of Addison's disease. **(FND)**

▶ Aspirin should be taken with food or milk to prevent gastric irritation. **(M-S)**

▶ During peritoneal dialysis, the nurse should observe the client for abdominal distention. **(M-S)**

▶ *Lanugo* is the fine, downy hair that commonly occurs on the body of a client with anorexia nervosa because of a loss of subcutaneous fat. **(PSY)**

▶ Extracorporeal shock wave lithotripsy is used to pulverize gallstones with shock waves. **(M-S)**

▶ If a pregnant client has candidiasis (*Candida albicans*) at the time of delivery, the neonate may develop thrush. **(MAT)**

▶ Ambulating the client is the best method to prevent postoperative respiratory complications. **(M-S)**

▶ If an umbilical cord continues to bleed even after being clamped, apply another clamp. **(MAT)**

▶ A fruity breath odor and Kussmaul's respirations are signs of diabetic ketoacidosis. **(M-S)**

▶ A sign of diabetic ketoacidosis is ketones, which are by-products of fat metabolism. Fat metabolism occurs when the body can't use glucose as an energy source and breaks down fat as a substitute. **(M-S)**

▶ Respiratory depression is a common fetal-neonatal adverse reaction to meperidine (Demerol) given within 2 hours of delivery. **(MAT)**

▶ Regular insulin is routinely given 30 minutes before meals. **(M-S)**

▶ The best indication that a mother is bonding with her baby is that she talks to the baby and touches him. **(MAT)**

▶ If the new mother is afraid to provide care to her neonate because she doesn't feel that she has the necessary skills, the nurse should provide the care by demonstrating the techniques to the mother and helping the mother provide the care. **(MAT)**

▶ If a neonate has symptoms of opioid withdrawal, the nurse should reduce environmental noises and stimulation. **(PED)**

▶ Signs of heroin withdrawal in the neonate include hyperactivity, irritability, and high-pitched crying. **(MAT)**

▶ Infantile anxiety is manifested by frequent crying. (PSY)

▶ According to the self-help group Alcoholics Anonymous, the first step toward recovering is admitting that you're an alcoholic and the first step in the treatment of alcoholism is detoxification. (PSY)

▶ Inflammation of the eyes is common in the person who recently smoked marijuana. (PSY)

▶ Although marijuana isn't known for its addictive qualities, use often leads to experimentation with other drugs, causes apathy, and suppresses motivation. (PSY)

▶ After the death of a loved one, the nurse should allow the family to spend time with the body. Doing so promotes the reality of the loss and allows the grieving process to begin. (FND)

▶ Urinary output is the best indication that a client with nephrotic syndrome is beginning to respond to corticosteroid therapy. (M-S)

▶ The best method to prevent blood clots after surgery is ambulation. (M-S)

▶ Adverse effects of aminophyllines include restlessness, irritability, tachycardia, hypertension, and insomnia. (M-S)

▶ The postmenopausal woman should perform breast self-examination on the same day each month, such as the 1st day of the month or the same day of the month as her birthday. (M-S)

▶ Antibiotics are ineffective in the treatment of viruses. (M-S)

▶ When the nurse must notify the physician of a change in a client's condition, the nurse should first assess the client so that she can provide accurate and complete information to the physician. (FND)

▶ Persistent use of a nasal decongestant can cause rebound phenomenon, which worsens the congestion. (M-S)

▶ A client who has a blood relative with breast cancer is at increased risk for the cancer. (M-S)

▶ In a client with benign fibrocystic disease, fibrocystic lesions that are observed on X-ray become larger and tender just before menses. (M-S)

▶ Cancerous tumors are usually irregularly shaped and don't move freely because they're attached to surrounding tissue. (M-S)

▶ A baseline mammogram should be performed between ages 35 and 39. Routine mammograms should be performed every 1 to 2 years between ages 40 and 49 and annually at age 50 and older. (M-S)

▶ As part of breast self-examination, a woman should observe her breasts for asymmetry by standing before a mirror with her bra removed and her arms above her head. (M-S)

▶ A woman should use the pads of the four fingertips to examine her breasts.
(M-S)

▶ One of the methods used to examine the breasts is to palpate each breast in small circles, moving from the outer margin toward the nipple.   (M-S)

▶ A client who's scheduled for a mammogram should be instructed not to use underarm deodorant, body powder, or ointment because these substances could cause an artifact in the film.   (M-S)

▶ The drug of choice to treat status epilepticus is diazepam (Valium) I.V. (M-S)

▶ Oral hygiene is very important for the client who's taking phenytoin (Dilantin).
(M-S)

▶ After a head injury, clear fluid in the ears (cerebrospinal fluid) suggests injury to the meninges.   (M-S)

▶ When a client with a possible head and neck injury must be moved, the nurse should immobilize the head and neck and move them together.   (M-S)

▶ A client who has a head injury should be placed in a supine position, with his head slightly elevated, to reduce intracranial pressure and promote venous return.   (M-S)

▶ The best indicator of increasing intracranial pressure is a deteriorating level of consciousness. Another indicator is abnormal pupillary response such as dilation when a light is shined into the eye.   (M-S)

▶ The client who's taking mannitol should have a catheter because the osmotic effect of the drug causes increased urination.   (M-S)

▶ Adverse effects associated with mannitol therapy include dehydration, electrolyte imbalance, and diarrhea.   (M-S)

▶ The primary nursing intervention for the child who's admitted to the hospital in a sickle cell crisis is relieving pain.   (PED)

▶ A child who's in a sickle cell crisis is susceptible to dehydration and should be offered favorite fluids, such as ice pops and gelatins.   (PED)

▶ If both parents have the sickle cell trait (both are heterozygous), there's a 25% chance that an offspring would be born with sickle cell disease.   (PED)

▶ An infant who has acquired immunodeficiency syndrome commonly has thrush, mouth sores, and severe diaper rash.   (PED)

▶ Atopic dermatitis may be an allergic reaction.   (M-S)

▶ The treatment for dermatitis is typically directed at relieving pruritus (itching).
(M-S)

▶ The most common colloid bath used to treat the irritated, itchy skin of an infant with eczema is a mixture of baking soda and cornstarch in tepid water. **(PED)**

▶ Abuse should be suspected if the child's injuries are inconsistent with his medical history and his wounds are in various stages of healing. **(PED)**

▶ When a child has a head injury, the parents should be instructed to assess the child for headaches and vomiting and to awaken the child every 4 hours to evaluate the difficulty in arousing the child. **(PED)**

▶ At age 5 to 6 months, an infant can sleep through the night, take one or two naps a day, and roll from stomach to back. **(PED)**

▶ The best site for assessing the pulse of a child age 5 or younger is the point of maximal impulse (apical pulse). **(PED)**

▶ The nurse should teach the parent to place the infant in an upright position and to use a rubber-tipped medicine dropper to administer oral medication. **(PED)**

▶ A child with hemophilia shouldn't be given products that contain aspirin. **(PED)**

▶ Elbow restraints should be used to restrain the upper extremities of an infant after repair of a cleft lip. **(PED)**

▶ A toddler is developing autonomy when he says "no" to his parents' requests more frequently. **(PED)**

▶ A child's fear and anxiety about a new procedure may be minimized by allowing him to handle the equipment, when appropriate. **(PED)**

▶ Painful procedures shouldn't be performed in the child's hospital room because the child may come to view the room as a "torture chamber." **(PED)**

▶ A sign of a child's severe reaction to prolonged hospitalization is ignoring his parents. **(PED)**

▶ To counter the effects of prolonged hospitalization, the nurse should encourage the parents to sleep in the child's room and participate in his care. **(PED)**

▶ A significant finding in assessing a parent's potential for child abuse is the fact that the parent was abused as a child. **(PED)**

▶ When treating a person who's accused of a "crime against nature," sexual abuse, or child abuse, the nurse should maintain a nonjudgmental attitude. **(PSY)**

▶ Allowing the mother to provide basic care for her neonate promotes bonding. **(MAT)**

▶ To leave room for other foods, a toddler shouldn't drink more than 24 ounces of milk each day. **(PED)**

▶ Noisy respirations indicate that a tracheostomy needs suctioning.   (M-S)

▶ Before suctioning the client, the nurse should provide 100% oxygen for 1 to 2 minutes.   (M-S)

▶ Wounds are cleaned from the center to the outer edges to prevent transferring microorganisms from outside to inside the wound.   (FND)

▶ Hearing aids amplify sound waves.   (FND)

▶ A client with a retinal detachment may see flashes of light and a veil-like curtain in the visual field.   (M-S)

▶ Medication isn't normally administered in bottle feedings because the infant may not drink the entire contents of the bottle.   (PED)

▶ A child who's in Bryant's traction shouldn't have a trapeze attached to the bed because the child must remain flat in bed.   (PED)

▶ In a pregnant woman, a positive urine test result for albumin indicates the need for further assessment.   (MAT)

▶ A pregnant client who's admitted to labor and delivery wouldn't normally receive an enema if she has vaginal bleeding.   (MAT)

▶ Decreasing blood pressure, increased pulse, and increased respirations are signs of impending shock in the postoperative client.   (M-S)

▶ After transurethral prostatic resection, the client should be encouraged to drink large amounts of fluid to keep urine diluted and prevent blood clots from forming in the urine and obstructing the catheter.   (M-S)

▶ If the client is fully dilated and her cervix is 100% effaced, she's entering the second stage of labor.   (MAT)

▶ One ounce is equal to 30 ml.   (FND)

▶ A rash may indicate a reaction to penicillin; therefore, the nurse should withhold the medication and notify the physician.   (M-S)

▶ To promote healthy elimination, adults should drink 1,500 ml of fluid daily and consume a regular diet that includes adequate amounts of fruits and vegetables.   (M-S)

▶ To minimize discomfort when administering an I.M. injection into the dorsogluteal site, the client should position his toes inward.   (FND)

▶ Before administering the influenza vaccine, the nurse should ask the client whether he's allergic to eggs or egg products.   (M-S)

▶ An adult client who has a high fever should receive 2,500 to 3,000 ml of fluid daily if he has no preexisting cardiovascular or kidney diseases.   (M-S)

▶ A tepid bath is used to limit body heat loss.   (FND)

▶ The nurse shouldn't ask a "yes or no" question (such as "Do you want to take your medicine?") unless she's prepared to accept the answer.　(FND)

▶ If the client begins to shiver or has chills, a tepid bath should be discontinued.　(FND)

▶ The nurse should report a fever in a client who's undergoing dialysis.　(M-S)

▶ A suprapubic cystostomy tube is surgically inserted directly into the bladder.　(M-S)

▶ Urine flow should be consistent with the client's routine urine output.　(M-S)

▶ An adult client who has urolithiasis should receive 2,500 ml of fluid daily, ambulate frequently, and have his urine strained to harvest calculi.　(M-S)

▶ To reduce discomfort during extracorporeal shock wave lithotripsy, the client is given medication before the procedure. The lower half of the body is usually submerged in water or the client's lower body is surrounded by fluid-filled bags.　(M-S)

▶ Clients who have benign prostatic hyperplasia typically have nocturia, hesitation on urination, a decreased urinary stream, and dribbling.　(M-S)

▶ Fertilization usually occurs in the fallopian tubes.　(MAT)

▶ The size of a woman's breasts has no effect on her ability to breast-feed or to provide adequate nutrition for her nursing infant.　(MAT)

▶ The size of the true pelvis in comparison to the size of the fetus's head (cephalopelvic ratio) is one factor that may determine whether the mother can deliver vaginally.　(MAT)

▶ A 3- to 4-month-old infant in a prone position should be able to lift his head 45 to 90 degrees.　(PED)

▶ If the infant pushes medication out of his mouth because of the extrusion reflex, the nurse should scoop it up and return it to the infant's mouth.　(PED)

▶ New foods should be introduced to the 4- or 5-month-old infant one food at a time, about 1 week apart, to identify food allergies.　(PED)

▶ Carotenosis is occasionally seen in infants who are fed orange vegetables such as carrots.　(PED)

▶ Home water heaters shouldn't be set above 120° F (48.9° C).　(FND)

▶ A high concentration of oxygen administered to the premature neonate can cause retrolental fibroplasia and blindness.　(PED)

▶ Bladder training is usually easier to accomplish than bowel training and should be started at age 18 to 24 months.　(PED)

▶ In an adolescent, telltale signs of suicidal intention include loss of a significant friend, loss of a friend to suicide, a change in appearance, decreased interest in activities that formerly brought pleasure, loss of interest in school, increased substance abuse, suicide notes, fascination with death, decreased appetite, and changes in hygiene. **(PSY)**

▶ In treating the child with impetigo, local and systemic antibiotics are usually used concomitantly and fingernails are trimmed to prevent scratching. **(PED)**

▶ The best position for lumbar puncture in a child is the side-lying position, with the knees drawn up. **(PED)**

▶ Air that leaks into surrounding tissue at the insertion site of a chest tube can cause subcutaneous emphysema. **(M-S)**

▶ The client should void before having a pelvic examination. **(M-S)**

▶ Breakthrough bleeding often occurs during the early phase of oral contraceptive use. **(MAT)**

▶ A woman shouldn't douche for several days before a Papanicolaou test. **(M-S)**

▶ The client should be instructed to perform breast self-examination while taking a shower. **(M-S)**

▶ A blood pressure cuff bladder should cover at least two-thirds of the limb at its midpoint and should be as wide as 40% of the midlimb circumference. **(FND)**

▶ The organ that usually sustains damage from hypertension is the eye. **(M-S)**

▶ Administration of diuretics in the morning minimizes disruption of sleep for urination. **(M-S)**

▶ Cholesterol is animal fat that attaches to the intimal layer of arteries. It enlarges to form plaque that occludes the passageway of the vessels, causing atherosclerosis. **(M-S)**

▶ An adverse effect of nicotinic acid tablets that are used to lower triglyceride levels is flushing of the skin. **(M-S)**

▶ Adverse effects of colestipol (Colestid), an antihyperlipidemic drug, are constipation and abdominal pain and distention. **(M-S)**

▶ A stress electrocardiogram should be stopped if the client has chest pain, dangerous cardiac rhythm changes, or a significant increase in blood pressure. **(M-S)**

▶ Adverse effects of nitroglycerin tablets include headache, flushing, and dizziness. **(M-S)**

▶ If a food has 4 g of protein, 28 g of fat, and 62 g of carbohydrates, the number of calories is 516. Protein and carbohydrates each have 4 calories/gram, and fat has 9 calories/gram. **(FND)**

▶ Dizziness and vertigo are common adverse effects of the vasodilating drug isosorbide (Isordil), which is used in the prolonged treatment of angina. These effects may be minimized by reducing the dosage or instructing the client to take the medication at night, before going to sleep. **(M-S)**

▶ The best nursing intervention for the anxious client commonly is to simply allow the client to express his anxiety. **(PSY)**

▶ In communicating with the anxious client, the nurse should use short, simple sentences. **(PSY)**

▶ Avoidance is the most common defense mechanism used by clients who have a phobia. **(PSY)**

▶ *Art therapy* is a therapeutic technique that may help a person share a thought that's too painful to discuss. **(PSY)**

▶ Any person who survives a catastrophic event or a very unusual experience is at risk for posttraumatic stress disorder. **(PSY)**

▶ Unless otherwise directed, the solution used to irrigate an indwelling urinary catheter is normal saline. **(FND)**

▶ A characteristic of obstructive jaundice is dark brown urine. **(M-S)**

▶ Dark urine occurs when bilirubin is excreted by the kidneys instead of the intestinal tract. **(M-S)**

▶ For the client with osteoporosis, the desired safety outcome is preventing injuries from falls. **(FND)**

▶ Before a bolus feeding is given through a gastric tube, the residual stomach contents should be checked. Gastric feedings are held if more than 100 ml remains from the previous feeding. **(M-S)**

▶ After a gastric feeding, the gastric tube should be irrigated with water and the head of the bed should be elevated. **(FND)**

▶ Clients who have gastric ulcers usually report that their discomfort goes away after they eat. **(M-S)**

▶ A positive result on a fecal occult blood test indicates bleeding in the GI tract. **(M-S)**

▶ Clients who have peptic ulcers are given antibiotics, such as tetracycline, to eliminate *Helicobacter pylori*, bacteria that deplete gastric mucus. **(M-S)**

▶ Signs of a perforated ulcer include abdominal rigidity and pain. **(M-S)**

▶ To confirm the proper placement of a gastric sump tube, the nurse should instill a bolus of air and then listen for a whooshing sound.   (FND)

▶ To ensure that a client performs the postoperative procedures that are necessary for recovery, the nurse should first alleviate pain by teaching the client techniques for positioning, splinting, or controlled breathing or by administering prescribed analgesics.   (M-S)

▶ Water that's used to irrigate a gastric tube should be recorded as intake on the intake and output record.   (FND)

▶ A client who's at risk for dumping syndrome should be taught to consume a diet that's low in carbohydrates and to avoid fluids during meals.   (M-S)

▶ After a partial gastrectomy, the client should be taught to eat small meals and to lie down for a short period after eating to delay gastric emptying.   (M-S)

▶ Absence of free hydrochloric acid suggests stomach cancer.   (M-S)

▶ When inserting a nasogastric tube preoperatively, the nurse should ask the client to place his chin on his chest. This position facilitates passage of the tube down the esophagus and away from the trachea.   (FND)

▶ Low intermittent suction is best for single-lumen nasogastric tubes.   (FND)

▶ Low continuous suction is best for vented, or double-lumen, nasogastric tubes.   (FND)

▶ A client who's undergoing nasogastric suctioning should receive nothing by mouth. The fluid that's instilled will be suctioned out of the stomach, further depleting the electrolytes and causing an imbalance.   (FND)

▶ There are 1,000 mcg in 1 mg.   (FND)

▶ There are 62.5 mg in 1 grain.   (FND)

▶ Concentrated urine is one of the first signs of dehydration.   (M-S)

▶ A *trochanter roll* is used to maintain the hip in a neutral position and prevent external rotation.   (FND)

▶ One teaspoon equals 5 ml; 1 tablespoon equals 15 ml.   (FND)

▶ When administering solid medication and cough syrup at the same sitting, the nurse should administer the cough syrup last.   (FND)

▶ To aid in expectoration of pulmonary secretions, fluid intake should be increased to thin secretions.   (M-S)

▶ After obtaining a sputum specimen, the nurse should provide oral hygiene care.   (FND)

▶ The most common characteristic of pleurisy is a sharp, stabbing pain on inspiration.   (M-S)

▶ Genital warts caused by human papillomavirus are associated with the development of cancer in the vulva, vagina, and cervix. (M-S)

▶ The client should use a condom that contains the spermicide nonoxynol 9 to reduce the spread of human immunodeficiency virus. (M-S)

▶ Oral contraceptives are best taken at about the same time each day, preferably in the evening. (M-S)

▶ In a client who's taking oral contraceptives, smoking increases the risk of blood clots. (M-S)

▶ After a vasectomy, the client should use an additional method of birth control for 6 weeks. The sperm count should be zero before the client considers himself sterile. (M-S)

▶ Complications of percutaneous transluminal coronary angioplasty include chest pain, abnormal cardiac rhythms, and bleeding from the operative site. (M-S)

▶ Bleeding is the most common adverse reaction associated with thrombolytic drug therapy. (M-S)

▶ The best method to open the airway of an unconscious client is the chin lift and head tilt. (M-S)

▶ After successful cardiopulmonary resuscitation, the nurse should place the client in a side-lying position. (M-S)

▶ A sudden increase in energy in the pregnant client is associated with the "nesting instinct" and indicates approaching labor. (MAT)

▶ During the latent phase of the first stage of labor, the pregnant client is encouraged to drink fluids to prevent dehydration. (MAT)

▶ The fetal heart rate should be assessed every 30 minutes during the latent phase of labor, every 15 minutes during the active phase, and every 5 minutes during the transition phase. (MAT)

▶ Epidural anesthesia can be performed at any point during labor; however, it's usually given when the primigravida is dilated 5 to 6 cm and the multigravida is dilated 3 to 4 cm. (MAT)

▶ In assessing uterine contractions, the nurse should palpate the fundus of the uterus, just above the umbilicus, because the contractions are strongest at this location. (MAT)

▶ After the rupture of membranes, the client's temperature should be assessed every hour because of the increased risk of infection. (MAT)

▶ An episiotomy prevents lacerations and damage to the perineum and speeds the delivery process. (MAT)

▶ To insert a vaginal suppository, the client should be in a lithotomy position, with her knees flexed.   (MAT)

▶ Vaginal suppositories are best administered at bedtime; a recumbent position aids in retaining the medication.   (FND)

▶ Yeast is present in the intestinal tract and is spread into the vagina by wiping from the rectum to the vagina; therefore, the client should wipe from front to back.   (FND)

▶ Infertility is commonly caused by pelvic inflammatory disease.   (M-S)

▶ The nurse should walk behind and slightly to the side of the client who's using a walker.   (FND)

▶ The best time to perform postural drainage is in the morning.   (FND)

▶ The best way to prevent contractures is exercise.   (FND)

▶ After a myocardial infarction, nursing action is directed toward allowing the heart muscle to rest by providing bed rest, oxygen, pain relief, and a bedside commode.   (M-S)

▶ After cataract extraction, intraocular tension is minimized by encouraging the client to rest his eyes by using eye patches, avoid reading until it's approved by the physician, avoid straining to defecate, avoid bending at the waist, and avoid lying with the affected eye dependent.   (M-S)

▶ Kegel exercises, which strengthen the pubococcygeal muscles, can help to relieve stress incontinence.   (M-S)

▶ To determine whether a client is adapting to changes created by illness or injury, the nurse should assess whether he acknowledges the deficit and chooses a level of activity that challenges his physical and mental capabilities appropriately.   (FND)

▶ During a spinal tap, the client must remain motionless and avoid coughing.   (M-S)

▶ After a cholecystectomy, the nurse should clamp the T tube when the client eats.   (M-S)

▶ Exercising the legs helps prevent venous stasis and venous thrombosis. (M-S)

▶ Delirium tremens usually causes progressive deterioration of mental processes and orientation to person, place, and time.   (PSY)

▶ For the client with Alzheimer's disease, the room should be brightly lit during the daytime.   (M-S)

▶ If a client who's receiving an enema can't retain the fluid any longer, the nurse should clamp the tubing and instruct him to take deep breaths.   (FND)

▶ An elderly client has a decreased need for calories.   (M-S)

► Use of an over-the-bed trapeze is contraindicated for the client who has a ruptured lumbar disk. **(M-S)**

► The client shouldn't use makeup, including lipstick and powder, before surgery because it could interfere with visual assessment of the client. **(M-S)**

► In treating the burn patient, the most important concern is assessment of airway function. **(M-S)**

► To conserve the energy of the premature neonate, the nurse should cluster nursing care activities. **(PED)**

► After the insertion of tympanostomy tubes in the child, the parent should be instructed to have the child wear earplugs when bathing. **(PED)**

► The most common adverse effects of isoniazid are peripheral neuritis, hepatitis, and hypersensitivity. **(M-S)**

► In the client who's receiving isoniazid, aspartate aminotransferase and alanine aminotransferase levels should be monitored. **(M-S)**

► For the client with tuberculosis to be considered no longer infectious, results of sputum cultures on three consecutive mornings must be negative. **(M-S)**

► After a catheter is removed, dribbling may occur because of a weakened urinary sphincter. **(M-S)**

► Before administering meperidine (Demerol), which is a central nervous system depressant, the nurse should assess the client's respiratory status. **(M-S)**

► Tomato juice has a high amount of vitamin C, which promotes wound healing. **(FND)**

► When questioning a client, the nurse should proceed from general questions to specific questions. An example is "Are you experiencing any pain?" followed by "Could you tell me the location of your pain?" **(FND)**

► The first symptom of tracheal edema as a result of bronchoscopy-related trauma is dyspnea. **(M-S)**

► A chest tube is inserted to drain blood and other fluids and to reestablish and maintain negative pressure. **(M-S)**

► Risk factors for coronary artery disease include obesity, a diet that's high in saturated fats, and increasing amounts of stress. **(M-S)**

► During the immediate postamputation phase, pain medication is the treatment of choice. **(M-S)**

► If the client can communicate, the best source of information about a client's illness is the client himself. **(FND)**

► The goal of surgical preparation is to reduce the total number of bacteria. **(M-S)**

▶ If the client has no signs of dehydration but his oral mucous membranes are dry, he's breathing through his mouth instead of his nose.   (FND)

▶ A newly applied plaster cast normally dries within 24 hours and dries from the outside to the inside.   (FND)

▶ Aminophylline relaxes the smooth muscles of the bronchi and relieves bronchospasms.   (M-S)

▶ Before amniocentesis, the client should empty her bladder.   (MAT)

▶ Protein is restricted in clients who have severe renal impairment because they can't eliminate nitrogen, a waste product of protein metabolism.   (M-S)

▶ Vitamin D is known as the "sunshine vitamin."   (FND)

▶ Orange and green vegetables are the primary source of vitamin A.   (FND)

▶ Clothing that becomes wet in a mist (moist) tent should be changed.   (FND)

▶ The mist in a moist tent should never be so dense that it obstructs the view of the client's breathing pattern.   (FND)

▶ An infant with celiac disease can be given corn and rice products and Probana formula.   (PED)

▶ Night blindness is associated with vitamin A deficiency.   (FND)

▶ After liver biopsy, nursing care is directed at minimizing the risk of hemorrhage.   (M-S)

▶ If the client has incomplete emptying after a colostomy irrigation, the nurse should irrigate the colostomy with normal saline and suggest a morning evacuation.   (M-S)

▶ A neonate who has hydrocephalus should have his position changed every 1 to 2 hours.   (PED)

▶ When feeding the infant who has had repair of a cleft lip, the nurse should place the infant in an upright position to aid swallowing, burping, and retention of formula or breast milk.   (PED)

▶ Before putting antiembolism stockings on the client, the nurse should have the client lie down with the feet elevated for 20 to 30 minutes.   (FND)

▶ When performing gastric gavage, the nurse should place the client in an upright position to minimize reflux.   (FND)

▶ An enteric-coated tablet shouldn't be crushed; it's designed to be dissolved in the GI tract.   (M-S)

▶ A *percutaneous transluminal coronary angioplasty* is a nonsurgical procedure that compresses plaque against the coronary artery wall.   (M-S)

▶ To help a client with poor vision locate his food on the tray, the nurse should refer to times on a clock. For example, "Your potatoes are at 12 o'clock, your bread is at 3 o'clock, and your steak is at 6 o'clock." **(FND)**

▶ When weighing a client with anorexia nervosa, the nurse should have the client step backward onto the scale while guiding her to ensure her safety. **(M-S)**

▶ After administering ear medication in a child, the nurse should place the child in a side-lying position for 2 to 3 minutes to ensure that the medication reaches the middle ear and eardrum. **(PED)**

▶ Hyperpyrexia puts the child at an increased risk for seizures. **(M-S)**

▶ The treatment protocol for acute leukemia involves three phases: induction (the client receives chemotherapy), consolidation (modified course of chemotherapy), and maintenance (small doses of chemotherapy every 3 to 4 weeks. **(M-S)**

▶ Before attempting to teach the client any procedure or task, the nurse should assess the client's willingness to learn and his current level of knowledge. **(FND)**

▶ A 15% isotonic dehydration in an infant is considered severe; for an older child, 10% is considered severe. **(FND)**

▶ A cleansing enema is administered before a barium enema to facilitate visualization of the colon. **(FND)**

▶ Thiazides are potassium-depleting diuretics. A client who's taking them should increase his oral intake of potassium. **(M-S)**

▶ The nurse should report a prolonged clotting time to the physician; normally, slow clotting results in postponement of surgery. **(M-S)**

▶ Three cellular products that help the body fight infection or invasion are interferon, lymphokines, and interleukins. **(M-S)**

▶ The daily dose of digoxin is 0.125 to 0.5 mg daily. **(M-S)**

▶ Expect diuresis in 1 to 3 weeks in a child with nephrotic syndrome (nephrosis). **(M-S)**

▶ A sign that heart failure is resolving is increased urine output. **(M-S)**

▶ *Risk for body image disturbance* is a diagnosis for the female client with Cushing's syndrome. These clients are at risk for masculinization, or the development of male characteristics. **(M-S)**

▶ In the client with Graves' disease, the first indication of an impending thyroid crisis is an elevation of temperature over baseline. **(M-S)**

▶ A sign of Graves' disease (hyperthyroidism) is exophthalmus (bulging eyes). **(M-S)**

▶ A drug that's used to treat hyperthyroidism is propylthiouracil. (M-S)

▶ Propylthiouracil should be stored in a light-resistant container and taken at the prescribed time throughout the day (typically every 8 hours). (M-S)

▶ After a complete or partial parathyroidectomy, the client should consume a diet high in calcium. (M-S)

▶ Calcium gluconate and calcium chloride I.V. are the drugs of choice for treating tetany associated with hypothyroidism. (M-S)

▶ Bronzelike pigmentation of the skin is associated with Addison's disease. (M-S)

▶ Clients with Addison's disease should consume foods that are high in sodium, such as cheese, milk, and processed (canned) foods. (M-S)

▶ In the client with Addison's disease, extreme stress, salt depletion, infection, trauma, and extremes in temperature increase the risk of an addisonian crisis. (M-S)

▶ Addisonian crisis causes severe hypotension and requires the administration of I.V. cortisol. (M-S)

▶ A parathyroid tumor normally causes a shift of calcium from the bones to the blood and results in renal calculi and leg cramps. (M-S)

▶ A decrease in bone mass as a result of loss of calcium from the bones increases the risk of pathologic fractures. (M-S)

▶ The normal fetal heart rate is 120 to 160 beats/minute (including the rate during contractions). (MAT)

▶ In the 12th week of pregnancy, the fundus should be at the level of the symphysis pubis. (MAT)

▶ A pregnant client without any complications should be seen monthly for the first 28 weeks, every 2 weeks up to 36 weeks, and then weekly until delivery. (MAT)

▶ When lifting the client's legs to place them in the lithotomy position, the nurse should lift both legs at the same time to prevent a back injury. (FND)

▶ Signs of corneal transplant rejection include loss of vision, redness, and photosensitivity. (M-S)

▶ Even if a client who's taking interferon for multiple sclerosis has anorexia and nausea, the medication must be administered. The nurse should suggest smaller, more frequent meals. (M-S)

▶ Mirrors should be removed from the room of a client who has facial burns until he receives counseling about the disfigurement. (M-S)

▶ A consistent finding in clients who have multiple sclerosis is that hot weather and hot water increase weakness. (M-S)

▶ When injecting a medication into a client who received a previous injection, the nurse shouldn't use a site that's closer than 1" (2.5 cm) to a previous site. (FND)

▶ For I.M. injections in a small or medium-sized adult, a 1½" (3.8 cm) needle is the correct size. (FND)

▶ The mitral valve is located between the left atrium and the left ventricle. (FND)

▶ Clubbing of digits is seen in adults and children who have chronic cardiopulmonary diseases. (M-S)

▶ An elevated temperature, which inhibits and destroys pathogens, is the body's mechanism for fighting infections. (M-S)

▶ A sign of pericarditis is a friction rub, which has a grating or leathery sound. (M-S)

▶ Signs of diabetes insipidus are polyuria and a urine specific gravity of less than 1.005. (M-S)

▶ Skin traction pulls directly on the skin through the use of adhesive or elastic bandages. (FND)

▶ A sign of acromegaly is enlarged hands. (M-S)

▶ A water-deprivation test is used to aid in diagnosing diabetes insipidus; even when deprived of water, the kidneys can't concentrate urine. (M-S)

▶ During the oliguric phase of renal failure, the client is given fluid only equal to the amount of urine output. (M-S)

▶ When a client is on strict intake and output restriction, the amount of fluid permitted is distributed throughout the day (for example, 50% is given during the day shift, 30% during the evening shift, and 20% during the night shift). (FND)

▶ If a client who's in renal failure is administered a fluid challenge of 500 ml of I.V. fluids, he must be monitored for signs of heart failure and pulmonary edema. (M-S)

▶ If a client on fluid restriction is thirsty, hard candy may be used to provide a measure of relief. (M-S)

▶ An autistic child responds to his parents and others with indifference. (PED)

▶ Autistic children commonly display bizarre, repetitive body movements. (PED)

▶ The autistic child must be protected from self-harm, such as head banging and self-biting. **(PED)**

▶ The nurse should keep the environment of the autistic child consistent and should avoid changing routines. **(PED)**

▶ School-age children are usually told about medical procedures several days to a week before they occur. Toddlers are usually told just before the event occurs (normally no more than 1 day), and infants are told just as the event happens. **(PED)**

▶ Before discontinuing an indwelling urinary catheter that has been in place for an extended time, the nurse should clamp the tubing and allow the bladder to expand several times. **(FND)**

▶ A child who has croup shouldn't be given cough suppressants; suppressing the cough may worsen the child's respiratory status. **(PED)**

▶ Total parenteral nutrition solutions should be stored in the refrigerator and removed 30 to 60 minutes before delivery; chilled solution can cause hypothermia. **(FND)**

▶ The primary purpose of providing skin care at the insertion site of skeletal pins is to protect the bone from osteomyelitis. **(M-S)**

▶ Respiratory distress can be caused by fat embolism, which occurs 24 to 48 hours after the fracture of a long bone. **(M-S)**

▶ To break the suction of the nursing infant, the mother should insert her finger into the corner of the infant's mouth or gently press his chin downward. **(MAT)**

▶ After percutaneous bladder aspiration, the client's urine may be slightly pink; frank bleeding should be reported to the physician. **(M-S)**

▶ A Bradford frame is used for children who must be immobilized for a long time. **(PED)**

▶ *Beriberi disease,* which causes profound weakness, is a serious deficiency of vitamin B_1. **(M-S)**

▶ The nurse should use a Z-track method to administer injectable forms of iron. **(FND)**

▶ A client who receives an organ transplant must take an immunosuppressant drug for life. **(M-S)**

▶ A sign of congenital hip dislocation is an *Ortolani click,* which is heard on abduction of the neonate's leg on the affected side. **(PED)**

▶ Treatment for congenital hip dislocation is a Pavlik harness or the use of two or three diapers to maintain the leg in abduction. **(M-S)**

▶ Treatment for Ewing's tumor or sarcoma includes radiation and chemotherapy. Amputation usually isn't performed because cancer cells can spread via bone marrow. **(M-S)**

▶ Red tissue that blanches should be massaged, and preventive measures should be instituted to prevent an ulcer from forming. For example, the nurse should increase the frequency of turning, ensure an adequate diet, maintain a clean and dry bed, and prevent injuries caused by shearing force, friction, or pressure. **(M-S)**

▶ Signs of thalassemia major include pronounced bone hyperactivity, resulting in thickening of the cranium, and a Down syndrome appearance. **(M-S)**

▶ The neonate's head typically is 1" (2 to 3 cm) larger than his chest. **(MAT)**

▶ "Birds of a feather flock together" and "Don't cry over spilled milk" are examples of proverbs that are used to assess the client's abstract reasoning ability. **(PSY)**

▶ Abstract reasoning ability is compromised in schizophrenics, who commonly think in concrete terms. For example, the client with schizophrenia might interpret "people who live in glass houses shouldn't throw stones" as "the stones will break the glass." **(PSY)**

▶ Possible allergic reactions to iodine dye include dyspnea, sweating, nausea, vomiting, and chills. **(M-S)**

▶ The major complications of paracentesis are hypovolemia and shock as a result of fluid drainage and fluid shift. **(M-S)**

▶ Otitis media is common in the infant with a cleft palate. **(PED)**

▶ Signs and symptoms of malabsorption syndrome are weight loss, muscle wasting, bloating, and steatorrhea. **(M-S)**

▶ A client who's receiving chemotherapy is placed in reverse isolation. **(M-S)**

▶ A fever in the first 24 hours after delivery is commonly caused by dehydration rather than infection. **(MAT)**

▶ Two common manifestations of systemic lupus erythematosus are early morning stiffness and facial erythema that appears in a butterfly pattern. **(M-S)**

▶ Hypovolemia is the most common and most fatal complication of acute pancreatitis. **(M-S)**

▶ When instilling eye ointment and eyedrops into the same eye, the nurse should administer the eyedrops first. **(FND)**

▶ A child who has measles or chickenpox should be put in isolation. **(PED)**

▶ Greenstick fractures are the most common type of fractures in children. **(PED)**

▶ The nurse's role regarding a client's will is to record in his health record that he created a will and to document his current mental status. (FND)

▶ The infant's respiratory rate and apical pulse should be counted for 1 minute. (PED)

▶ A client with gastroesophageal reflux disease should be instructed to decrease his intake of fatty foods. (M-S)

▶ A tuning fork is used in the Rinne test or Weber's test to assess for sensory or conductive hearing loss. (M-S)

▶ The fulminating form of hepatitis resembles acute liver failure and may result in death. (M-S)

▶ Insulin promotes the conversion of fatty acids to fat, regulates the rate at which carbohydrates are used by cells for energy, and stimulates the synthesis of protein. (M-S)

▶ Delta hepatitis (hepatitis D) must coexist with hepatitis B. (M-S)

▶ Food and water intake aren't restricted before a thyroid function test. (M-S)

▶ If a client signs a consent form for a procedure and then makes a statement that suggests that he doesn't understand the procedure, therefore indicating that he isn't informed, the physician should be notified of the client's lack of understanding before the client receives preprocedure medication. (FND)

▶ Children with hepatitis are usually anicteric. (PED)

▶ A normal healthy stoma is bright red or pink; sustained dark coloration or paleness indicates compromised blood flow to the tissue. (M-S)

▶ A low-residue diet includes no fruits, vegetables, or whole grains or cereals. (FND)

▶ Alendronate (Fosamax) should be taken on an empty stomach. (M-S)

▶ After insertion of a Abbott-Miller intestinal tube, the client should be ambulated. (M-S)

▶ The best position for irrigating a stoma is sitting on a toilet. (FND)

▶ One of the best methods to detect fecal impaction is digital examination. (M-S)

▶ Carbonated beverages promote gas production and should be eliminated from the diet of the client who's prone to tympanites. (M-S)

▶ The primary purpose of a sitz bath is comfort. (FND)

▶ The most common form of cirrhosis of the liver in the United States is Laënnec's cirrhosis as a result of alcohol abuse. (M-S)

▶ Spider angiomas are seen in clients with Laënnec's cirrhosis and are manifested by central red bodies with radiating branches. **(M-S)**

▶ The bladder should be emptied before paracentesis. **(M-S)**

▶ Clients with Tourette syndrome tend to make uncontrollable audible sounds or utter obscenities. **(M-S)**

▶ A sign of cystic fibrosis is salty-tasting skin. **(M-S)**

▶ The typical postoperative diet is clear liquids for the first 24 hours. **(M-S)**

▶ To reduce the risk of paralytic ileus, the client who has had general anesthesia isn't given solid food until bowel sounds return. **(M-S)**

▶ A doll can be used as a teaching aid to help a preschooler understand a procedure. **(PED)**

▶ It's normal for a 4- or 5-year-old child to have an imaginary friend. **(PED)**

▶ The client who has systemic lupus erythematosus should remain in a calm environment, avoid exposure to the sun, and avoid the use of dusting powder. **(M-S)**

▶ Continuous bubbling is abnormal in a water-sealed chamber but normal in a suction-controlled chamber. **(FND)**

▶ Eyedrops are instilled in the lower conjunctival sac to prevent damaging the cornea. **(FND)**

▶ Constipation is an adverse reaction to antacids. **(M-S)**

▶ Hospice-care facilities provide care for terminally ill clients. **(FND)**

▶ Respite care provides temporary nursing care so that the primary caregiver has an opportunity to do other activities. **(FND)**

▶ Grunting on expiration, seesaw retractions, and nasal flaring are signs of respiratory distress in the infant. **(PED)**

▶ Liquid supplements should be offered between meals so that they don't replace meals. **(FND)**

▶ Before performing a procedure on an adult, and even before bringing the necessary equipment to the bedside, the nurse should explain what will occur. **(FND)**

▶ The first action to take in resuscitation is establishing or maintaining an airway. **(M-S)**

▶ A client who looks at or touches the affected area is showing acceptance of an alteration in body appearance. **(FND)**

▶ Dizziness, light-headedness, nausea, and vomiting are symptoms of supine hypotension syndrome, which is treated by having the client turn to his left side. The nurse should explain the cause so that the client can prevent a recurrence. **(M-S)**

▶ *Gravidity* is the number of pregnancies without regard to outcome. *Parity* is the number of pregnancies that reached viability (20+ weeks). Further clarification of obstetric data is made with the **F/TPAL** system:

– **F/T** indicates full-term delivery at 38+ weeks' gestation.

– **P** indicates preterm delivery between 20 and 37 weeks' gestation.

– **A** indicates abortion or loss of fetus before 20 weeks' gestation.

– **L** indicates the number of children living (if a child has died, further explanation is needed to clarify the discrepancy in numbers). **(MAT)**

▶ *Parity* doesn't refer to the number of viable fetuses delivered, only to the number of deliveries. **(MAT)**

▶ The recommended iron supplement for the pregnant client is 30 to 60 mg daily. **(MAT)**

▶ For early identification of genetic defects, chorionic villus sampling is performed at 8 to 12 weeks' gestation. **(MAT)**

▶ *Percutaneous umbilical blood sampling* is a procedure in which a blood sample is obtained from the umbilical cord to identify anemia, genetic defects, and blood incompatibility. **(MAT)**

▶ *Uterine atony* is failure of the uterus to remain firmly contracted; the major cause is a full bladder. **(MAT)**

▶ Before initiating feeding, the caregiver should burp the infant to expel air from the stomach. **(PED)**

▶ In clients with mastitis, most authorities strongly encourage continuing breast-feeding on both the affected and the unaffected side. **(MAT)**

▶ The ideal place to check skin turgor on the infant is on the abdomen. **(PED)**

▶ *Doll's eye movement* is the lag between head movement and eye movement. **(M-S)**

▶ The most desirable diet for the infant up to age 6 months is breast milk. **(PED)**

▶ When assessing whether an infant is ready for the addition of solids to his diet, the nurse should look for the following indicators: the infant has doubled his birth weight, the infant demands 8 to 10 feedings in a 24-hour period, the infant drinks more than 1 qt of formula or breast milk daily, and the infant always seems hungry. **(PED)**

▶ Solids are introduced to the infant in the following order: rice cereal, fruits, oatmeal, prepared vegetables, and meat. **(PED)**

▶ The hepatitis B vaccine is given within 48 hours of birth. **(MAT)**

▶ Hepatitis B immune globulin is given within 12 hours of birth. **(MAT)**

▶ *HELLP syndrome* is an unusual variation of pregnancy-induced hypertension; the acronym stands for hemolysis, elevated liver enzymes, and low platelets. **(MAT)**

▶ Maternal serum alpha-fetoprotein is detectable at 7 weeks' gestation and peaks in the third trimester. High levels detected between the 16th and 18th weeks are associated with neural-tube defects. **(MAT)**

▶ An arrest of descent occurs when the fetus doesn't descend through the pelvic cavity during labor. It's commonly associated with cephalopelvic disproportion, and cesarean intervention is required. **(MAT)**

▶ *Third spacing* of fluid is a shifting of fluid from the intravascular space to the interstitial space, where it remains. **(FND)**

▶ *Thought broadcasting* is a type of delusion in which the person believes that his thoughts are being broadcast for the world to hear. **(PSY)**

▶ A client who's taking griseofulvin should maintain a high-fat diet, which enhances the secretion of bile. **(M-S)**

▶ Foods that are high in protein decrease the absorption of levodopa. **(M-S)**

▶ Cottage cheese, cream cheese, yogurt, and sour cream are permitted in the diet of a client who's taking a monoamine oxidase inhibitor for depression. **(PSY)**

▶ Normal central venous pressure is 2 to 8 mm Hg or 5 to 10 cm H_2O. **(M-S)**

▶ A decrease in central venous pressure indicates a decrease in circulating fluid volume, as is seen in shock. **(M-S)**

▶ An increase in central venous pressure is associated with an increase in circulating fluid volume, as is seen in renal failure. **(M-S)**

▶ If a central venous pressure reading must be obtained when the client is on a ventilator, the reading should be taken at the end of the expiratory cycle. **(M-S)**

▶ To ensure an accurate baseline central venous pressure reading, the zero point of the transducer must be at the level of the right atrium. **(M-S)**

▶ In Mönckeberg's arteriosclerosis, calcium deposits occur in the medial layer of the arterial walls. **(M-S)**

▶ Creatine kinase (CK)-MB, an isoenzyme of CK that's specific to the heart, increases 4 to 6 hours after a myocardial infarction, peaks at 12 to 18 hours, and returns to normal in 3 to 4 days. **(M-S)**

▶ A client who survives a myocardial infarction and has no other cardiopathology usually requires 6 to 12 weeks for a full recovery. **(M-S)**

▶ Risk factors associated with embolism are increased blood viscosity, decreased circulation, prolonged bed rest, and increased blood coagulability. **(M-S)**

▶ Sexual intercourse with a known partner usually can be resumed 4 to 8 weeks after a myocardial infarction. **(M-S)**

▶ A client who's recovering from a myocardial infarction should avoid eating or drinking alcoholic beverages before engaging in sexual intercourse. **(M-S)**

▶ *Dependent edema* is an early sign of right-sided heart failure. It's seen in the legs, where increased capillary hydrostatic pressure overwhelms plasma protein and causes a shift of fluid from the capillary beds to the interstitial spaces. **(M-S)**

▶ After supratentorial surgery, the client should have the head of the bed elevated 30 degrees. **(M-S)**

▶ An acid or ash diet acidifies urine. **(M-S)**

▶ Vitamin C and cranberry juice acidify urine. **(FND)**

▶ The client who's taking probenecid with colchicine for gout should take the medication with food. **(M-S)**

▶ If wound dehiscence is suspected, the nurse should examine the wound, monitor the vital signs, and report concerns or abnormal findings to the physician. **(M-S)**

▶ Miotics, such as pilocarpine, are administered to the client who has acute angle-closure glaucoma to increase the outflow of aqueous humor. **(M-S)**

▶ Zoster immune globulin is administered to stimulate immunity to varicella. **(M-S)**

▶ The most common symptoms associated with compartmental syndrome are pain that isn't relieved by analgesics, loss of movement, loss of sensation, pain with passive movement, and lack of pulse. **(M-S)**

▶ To help relieve muscle spasms in the client with multiple sclerosis, the nurse should administer baclofen (Lioresal) as ordered, assist the client with a warm soothing bath, and teach him progressive relaxation techniques. **(M-S)**

▶ The client who has a cervical spine injury and impairment at C5 can lift his shoulders and elbows partially but has no sensation below the clavicle. Respiration isn't impaired. **(M-S)**

▶ The client who has a cervical spine injury and impairment at C6 can lift his shoulders, elbows, and wrists partially but has no sensation below the clavicle, except for a small amount in his arms and thumbs.   (M-S)

▶ The client who has a cervical spine injury and impairment at C7 can lift his shoulders, elbows, wrists, and hands partially but has no sensation below mid-chest.   (M-S)

▶ Injuries to the spinal cord at C3 and above may be fatal because of a loss of innervation to the diaphragm and intercostal muscles.   (M-S)

▶ For every client problem, there's a nursing diagnosis; for every nursing diagnosis, there's an outcome; and for every outcome, there are interventions designed to make the outcome a reality. The key to answering NCLEX questions correctly is to identify the problem presented, formulate an outcome for that specific problem, and then select the intervention that will allow the client to reach that specific outcome.   (FND)

▶ Signs of meningeal irritation, as seen in meningitis, include nuchal rigidity, a positive Brudzinski's sign, and a positive Kernig's sign.   (M-S)

▶ Laboratory values that indicate bacterial pneumomeningitis include elevated cerebrospinal fluid protein level (greater than 100 mg/dl), decreased cerebrospinal fluid glucose level (less than 40 mg/dl), and increased white blood cell count (100 to 10,000/µl).   (M-S)

▶ To promote rest in the young child in a hospital setting, the first nursing action is to decrease environmental stimulation.   (PED)

▶ Before magnetic resonance imaging, the client should remove all objects containing metal, such as watches, bras, and jewelry.   (M-S)

▶ Normally, food and medicine aren't restricted before magnetic resonance imaging.   (M-S)

▶ A client who's undergoing magnetic resonance imaging lies supine on a padded table that moves through an imager.   (M-S)

▶ A client who's undergoing magnetic resonance imaging should be informed that he can ask questions during the procedure; however, he should be reminded that he may be asked to lie still at certain times.   (M-S)

▶ If contrast medium is used during magnetic resonance imaging, the client may experience diuresis when the medium is flushed from his body.   (M-S)

▶ Hepatitis C is spread primarily through blood (posttransfusion or in people who work with blood products), personal contact and, possibly, the fecal-oral route.   (M-S)

▶ The best wound soak for an open, infected, draining wound is a hot-moist dressing.   (M-S)

▶ To confirm the diagnosis of tuberculosis, a sputum culture is performed.
(M-S)

▶ Dexamethasone (Decadron) is a steroidal anti-inflammatory drug that's used to treat adrenal insufficiency. (M-S)

▶ During the first 24 hours after amputation, the residual limb is elevated on a pillow; after that time, the limb is placed flat to reduce the risk of hip flexion contracture. (M-S)

▶ A tourniquet should be in plain view at the bedside of the client who has an amputation. (M-S)

▶ An emergency tracheostomy set should be kept at the bedside of the client with suspected epiglottiditis. (M-S)

▶ The key word to use when reporting suspected cases of child abuse to the appropriate authorities is "suspected." (PED)

▶ The client who has acquired immunodeficiency syndrome shouldn't share a razor or a toothbrush; however, there are no special precautions for dinnerware or laundry. (M-S)

▶ Estriol level is used to assess fetal well-being, maternal renal functioning, and pregnancies that are complicated by diabetes. (MAT)

▶ Water that accumulates in a ventilator tube should be removed. (M-S)

▶ A symptom of sensory overload is a feeling of distress and hyperarousal accompanied by impaired thinking and concentration. (PSY)

▶ *Sensory deprivation* is a state in which overall sensory input is decreased.
(PSY)

▶ Sensory deprivation leads to daydreaming, inactivity, sleeping excessively, and reminiscing. (PSY)

▶ After total knee replacement surgery, the client's knee is kept in maximum extension for 3 days. (M-S)

▶ *Sjögren's syndrome* is a chronic inflammatory disorder that's associated with a decrease in salivation and lacrimation. It causes dryness of the mouth, eyes, and vagina. (M-S)

▶ The three brain barriers are the blood-brain barrier, blood–cerebrospinal fluid barrier, and brain–cerebrospinal fluid barrier. (M-S)

▶ Normal ranges and values of cerebrospinal fluid include the following: protein, 15 to 45 mg/100 ml; glucose (fasting), 50 to 75 mg/100 ml; red blood cell count, 0; white blood cell count, 0 to 4/µl; pH, 7.3; and potassium ions, 2.9 mmol/L. (M-S)

▶ A sign of Paget's disease is bowleggedness. (M-S)

▶ The following mnemonic can be used to determine whether a cranial nerve is a motor nerve:

I,	II,	III,	IV,	V,	VI,	VII,	VIII,	IX,	X,	XI,	XII
Some	Say	Marry	Money,	But	My	Brother	Says	Bad	Business	Marry	Money.

Here's how to interpret the mnemonic: If the word begins with an S, it indicates a sensory nerve; if it starts with an M, it indicates a motor nerve; if it starts with a B, it indicates both a sensory and a motor nerve. **(M-S)**

▶ The Glasgow Coma Scale, on which the client can obtain a score of 3 to 15, is used to evaluate the client's level of consciousness, pupil reaction, and motor activity. **(M-S)**

▶ Passive range-of-motion exercises are usually started 24 hours after a stroke and are performed four times daily. **(M-S)**

▶ The medical management goal in treating a client with a transient ischemic attack is to prevent a stroke. The client is given antihypertensive drugs, antiplatelet drugs or aspirin and, in some cases, warfarin (Coumadin). **(M-S)**

▶ A client who has an intraperitoneal shunt should be observed for increased abdominal girth. **(M-S)**

▶ In determining acid-base problems, the nurse should first note the pH. If it's above 7.45, it's a problem of alkalosis; if it's below 7.35, it's a problem of acidosis. Next, look at the partial pressure of arterial carbon dioxide ($Paco_2$). This is the respiratory indicator. If the pH is acidic and the $Paco_2$ is acidic (greater than 45 mm Hg), there's a match. The source of the problem is respiration, and the client has respiratory acidosis. If the pH is alkaline and the $Paco_2$ is also alkaline (less than 35 mm Hg), there's a match. The source of the problem is respiration, and the client has respiratory alkalosis. If the $Paco_2$ is normal, look at the bicarbonate (HCO_3^-), which is the metabolic indicator, and note whether it's acidic (less than 22 mEq/L) or alkaline (greater than 26 mEq/L). See which value the pH matches to determine whether the problem is metabolic acidosis or metabolic alkalosis. If both the $Paco_2$ and HCO_3^- are abnormal, the body is compensating. If the pH has returned to normal and the $Paco_2$ or HCO_3^- is still normal, the body is in full compensation. **(M-S)**

▶ The Tensilon (edrophonium) test is used to confirm myasthenia gravis. **(M-S)**

▶ A masklike facial expression is a sign of myasthenia gravis and Parkinson's disease. **(M-S)**

▶ For the client who follows Jewish custom, dairy and meat shouldn't be served at the same meal. (For instance, the client shouldn't be served a cheeseburger). **(FND)**

▶ The nurse shouldn't permit smoking, use an aerosol spray, or shake bed sheets around a client who has a tracheostomy. **(M-S)**

▶ The best way to prevent disuse osteoporosis is to ambulate the client. **(M-S)**

▶ Treatment for bleeding esophageal varices includes vasopressin, esophageal tamponade, iced saline lavage, and vitamin K. **(M-S)**

▶ Pheochromocytoma is a catecholamine-secreting neoplasm of the adrenal medulla that causes excessive production of epinephrine and norepinephrine. **(M-S)**

▶ Pheochromocytoma causes vision disturbances, headaches, hypertension, and elevated blood glucose levels. Clients with this condition should avoid caffeine. **(M-S)**

▶ The client shouldn't consume products that contain caffeine, such as cola, coffee, or tea, for at least 8 hours before obtaining a 24-hour urine sample for vanillylmandelic acid. **(M-S)**

▶ The best method to debride a wound is to use a wet-to-dry dressing. The dressing should be removed after it dries. **(M-S)**

▶ A client with an above-the-knee amputation should be placed in a prone position twice daily to prevent hip flexion contractures. **(M-S)**

▶ The nurse shouldn't place anything, including a thermometer, into the mouth of the child with suspected epiglottiditis. **(M-S)**

▶ Signs of hip dislocation are uneven leg lengths and external rotation of one leg. **(M-S)**

▶ In the client with Parkinson's disease, extrapyramidal syndrome is most likely caused by a deficiency of dopamine in the substantia nigra of the brain. **(M-S)**

▶ Immediate care of a full-thickness skin graft in the client with burns includes covering the site with a bulky dressing. **(M-S)**

▶ The donor site of a skin graft should be left exposed to the air. **(M-S)**

▶ Leaking around a T tube should be reported to the physician immediately. **(M-S)**

▶ Diphtheria is characterized by a pseudomembranous patch that covers the posterior pharynx. **(M-S)**

▶ A sign of tinea capitis in the child is a scratch on the scalp. **(PED)**

▶ Kwell shampoo for head lice is effective if there are no lice in the hair and no eggs (nits) attached to the hair shafts. **(M-S)**

▶ In the client with a Steinmann pin in the femur, adverse signs include erythema, edema, and pain around the pin site. **(M-S)**

▶ Signs of acute narrow-angle glaucoma include seeing halos around lights and having cloudy vision. **(M-S)**

▶ The client with a transection at C3 needs positive ventilation to survive the injury. **(M-S)**

▶ The nurse should keep the sac of myelomeningocele moist with normal saline solution. **(MAT)**

▶ After supratentorial surgery, the client should be placed in the semi-Fowler position. **(M-S)**

▶ After a tonsillectomy or an adenoidectomy, frequent swallowing may indicate excessive bleeding or hemorrhage. **(PED)**

▶ Women with diabetes mellitus tend to have varying levels of hyperglycemia and have large but physically immature infants. **(MAT)**

▶ Compared with the preoperative findings, the stress of surgery and anesthesia may cause a slight decrease in blood pressure and temperature and a slight increase in respiration. **(M-S)**

▶ Before helping a client with a urinary drainage bag to ambulate, the nurse should empty the bag. **(M-S)**

▶ If a client feels faint or dizzy during ambulation, he should immediately sit. **(FND)**

▶ When helping a client to ambulate, for safety the nurse shouldn't allow the client to put his arms around her shoulders. **(FND)**

▶ A cane should be carried 6 inches from the body, on the unaffected side, and advanced with the affected extremity. **(FND)**

▶ The three stages of generalized adaptation syndrome are alarm, resistance, and exhaustion (ARE). **(FND)**

▶ To prevent the formation of pressure ulcers, a client should be repositioned at least every 2 hours. **(FND)**

▶ A sterile object is no longer considered sterile if it comes in contact with an unsterile object or if it's moved out of the sterile field. **(FND)**

▶ The best administration schedule for around-the-clock antibiotic therapy is 6 a.m., 12 p.m., 6 p.m., and 12 a.m. **(FND)**

▶ A client who has a seizure disorder shouldn't take a bath because of the risk of drowning during a seizure. The nurse should suggest a shower instead. **(M-S)**

▶ The nurse should remove her gloves by turning them inside out. **(FND)**

▶ The nurse should adjust sterile gloves after both gloves are on. **(FND)**

▶ An increased lymphocyte count indicates bacterial or viral infection. **(M-S)**

▶ Vasoconstriction is the body's first adaptive response to injury. **(M-S)**

▶ The type of drainage expected from an infected wound is purulent. It tends to have a thicker consistency, with various colors specific to the type of organism, and may have an unpleasant odor.   (M-S)

▶ Mild anxiety causes a slight arousal state that enhances perception, learning, and productivity.   (FND)

▶ The primary method of preventing the spread of microorganisms in the hospital setting is proper hand washing for approximately 10 to 15 seconds.   (FND)

▶ The best diversional activity to meet the developmental needs of a 12-year-old boy who's in traction is to have friends visit him.   (PED)

▶ For a client who has somnambulism (sleepwalking), the most important nursing goal is to prevent injury by providing a safe environment.   (PED)

▶ *Empathy* is a style of communication that indicates that the listener understands the speaker's message and understands how he feels.   (FND)

▶ *Histamine* is the chemical that's released during an inflammatory response.   (FND)

▶ The *pain threshold*, or pain sensation, is the initial point at which the client feels pain.   (FND)

▶ After surgery for glaucoma, the head of the client's bed is elevated to the semi-Fowler position or as ordered to promote drainage of aqueous humor. (M-S)

▶ One difference between acute pain and chronic pain is its duration. Acute pain lasts less than 6 months, whereas chronic pain lasts longer than 6 months.   (FND)

▶ Clients whose fluid intake is restricted need frequent mouth care.   (FND)

▶ When washing dentures in a sink, the nurse should place a soft towel in the bottom of the sink to provide a cushion in case the dentures slip from her hands.   (FND)

▶ When providing oral care, the nurse should place an unconscious client on his side, with his head slightly lower than his body.   (FND)

▶ Candidiasis appears as a white to yellow curdlike substance that covers the affected area, such as mucous membranes of the mouth, vagina, uncircumcised penis, nails, and deep skin folds.   (M-S)

▶ Because nystatin is poorly absorbed in the mouth, to maximize its effect the client should swish the medication for 2 to 3 minutes in his mouth before swallowing.   (M-S)

▶ The higher nursing priority in treating a client with chemical injury to the eye is irrigation of sterile normal saline to remove the chemical from the eye.   (M-S)

▶ *Presbyopia* is impaired accommodation, and *hyperopia* is farsightedness secondary to aging. (M-S)

▶ When ambulating a blind client, the nurse should allow the client to hold her arm as she walks slightly ahead of him. (M-S)

▶ Mydriatics, such as atropine, are used to block sphincter muscle response to dilate the pupil. (M-S)

▶ If a client has retinal detachment in one eye, the nurse should cover both of the client's eyes with sterile patches to prevent further detachment. (M-S)

▶ Noisy respirations, dyspnea, and increased pulse and respirations indicate that a tracheostomy needs suctioning. (M-S)

▶ After bronchoscopy, fluids and food are withheld until the gag reflex returns. (M-S)

▶ Medication shouldn't be given in a bottle of formula or milk because the infant may not complete the feeding. (PED)

▶ The initial postoperative diet is usually clear liquid. The diet is then advanced as tolerated. (FND)

▶ Digital examination is performed to confirm the presence of hard, dry feces in the rectum. (FND)

▶ Paraphrasing a client's statement is a therapeutic communication technique that lets the client know that his message was heard and how it was interpreted. (FND)

▶ Constipation is an adverse effect of antacids that contain aluminum and calcium. (M-S)

▶ The most reliable test to determine the presence of human immunodeficiency virus in infants and small children is the immunoglobulin A test. (PED)

▶ When a client can't cough or produce sputum, and sputum is impairing the airway, suctioning is performed. (M-S)

▶ Before undergoing cardiac catheterization, a child should tour the catheterization laboratory or at least see pictures of the equipment. This type of preparation isn't necessary for young clients who will be anesthetized. (M-S)

▶ A sign of intracranial bleeding is altered level of consciousness. (M-S)

▶ Dark brown urine is a sign of obstructive jaundice. (M-S)

▶ Milk and other animal products are high in protein. (FND)

▶ The treatment for a client who has hypothyroidism and tetany is calcium gluconate or calcium chloride. (M-S)

▶ *Ecchymosis* occurs when small blood vessels rupture and bleed into the skin. (FND)

▶ When wrapping a lower extremity with a roller bandage, the nurse should start at the metatarsals and advance up the foot and leg.   (FND)

▶ To bandage a cone-shaped body part, the nurse should use a spiral reverse technique.   (FND)

▶ If permission to treat a minor is provided over the telephone, at least two people should hear the verbal consent.   (FND)

▶ When helping a client to move from a bed to a chair, the nurse should place the chair parallel to the bed and on the client's stronger side.   (FND)

▶ The first sign of compartment syndrome is sharp pain.   (M-S)

▶ Allowing a cast to dry using natural evaporation is the best method.   (M-S)

▶ To promote even drying of a plaster cast, a client should be turned frequently during the first 24 to 48 hours.   (M-S)

▶ A cast dries from the outside in. Therefore, a cast may be wet but appear dry.   (M-S)

▶ A fractured bedpan facilitates elimination by raising the buttocks slightly.   (FND)

▶ The most common source of an odor emitting from a cast is an infected wound.   (M-S)

▶ Bone cancer typically metastasizes to the lungs.   (M-S)

▶ A client who has a herniated disk should be rolled from side to side to maintain correct body alignment.   (M-S)

▶ Symptoms of varicose veins include aching, tiredness, and heaviness in the leg.   (M-S)

▶ Stasis ulcers are darkly pigmented, dry, and scaly.   (M-S)

▶ The formation of pink granulation tissue is a sign that a wound is healing.   (FND)

▶ The body part distal to a blood clot, or thrombus, usually is edematous because of interrupted venous blood flow and redistribution of plasma to the interstitial space.   (M-S)

▶ If a blood clot is suspected, the nurse shouldn't massage the leg and shouldn't have the client ambulate.   (M-S)

▶ A sign of upper GI bleeding is black or tarry stools.   (M-S)

▶ Signs of phlebitis include tenderness, warmth, erythema, and edema. The vessel also may have a cordlike appearance.   (M-S)

▶ Characteristics of peripheral vascular disease are thick, hard nails and thin, shiny skin that has little hair growth.   (M-S)

▶ Clients who have peripheral arterial insufficiency commonly have intermittent claudication (pain on ambulation).   (M-S)

▶ Pain associated with Raynaud's disease usually affects only the hands and feet.   (M-S)

▶ The *Schilling test* is a 24-hour urine test that's used to confirm the diagnosis of pernicious anemia.   (M-S)

▶ *Remission* is halting of the disease progress and absence of signs or symptoms.   (FND)

▶ The presenting sign of mononucleosis is sore throat.   (M-S)

▶ The nurse should seek out a depressed client and initiate a one-on-one interaction.   (PSY)

▶ Hodgkin's disease causes painless, unilateral enlargement of lymph nodes, usually in the axillary area of the arm or on the side of the neck. It affects teenage males more than any other group.   (M-S)

▶ Skin that is being irradiated should be protected from the sun during irradiation.   (M-S)

▶ The treatment for polycythemia vera involves removal of blood by phlebotomy.   (M-S)

▶ The most common problem observed in bone marrow aspiration is bleeding.   (M-S)

▶ *Purpura* is a small hemorrhage in the skin and mucous membranes.   (FND)

▶ Hypotension is a serious reaction to blood transfusion.   (M-S)

▶ The nurse can use silence and active listening to promote interactions with a depressed client.   (FND)

▶ A major source of stress for a hospitalized toddler is separation anxiety.   (PED)

▶ A major developmental task during the first trimester is accepting the pregnancy.   (MAT)

▶ In a psychiatric setting, a client who has both a substance abuse problem and a major psychiatric disorder has a dual diagnosis.   (PSY)

▶ A client who's in the late stage of multiple myeloma should be protected against pathological fractures caused by osteoporosis.   (M-S)

▶ Tricyclic antidepressants, such as amitriptyline (Elavil), shouldn't be administered to a client who has acute angle-closure glaucoma, benign prostatic hyperplasia, or coronary artery disease.   (M-S)

▶ One benefit of breast milk over formula is the presence of maternal antibodies.   (MAT)

▶ On readmission to a mental health unit, the client's compliance with medication orders should be assessed.   (PSY)

▶ When chest percussion therapy is performed on a child, percussions (clapping) should be confined to the area around the rib cage.   (PED)

▶ Pulmonary embolism is characterized by a sudden, sharp, stabbing pain in the chest; dyspnea; decreased breath sounds; and crackles, or pleural friction rub on auscultation.   (M-S)

▶ Most poisonings in children younger than age 6 occur when the child takes a toxic substance, such as a liquid cleaning product or medication, orally.   (PED)

▶ The most common nutritional problem in children in the United States is obesity.   (PED)

▶ A clinical manifestation of cardiac tamponade is distention of the neck veins.   (M-S)

▶ To prevent further damage, vomiting shouldn't be induced in a client who has swallowed oven cleaner, drain cleaner, or kerosene.   (M-S)

▶ A brilliant red reflex excludes most serious defects of the cornea, aqueous chamber, lens, and vitreous chamber.   (M-S)

▶ Preschool children commonly stutter because their vocabulary is increasing more rapidly than their ability to produce words. This dysfluency is a common characteristic of language development.   (PED)

▶ In answering parents' questions about their child's condition, the nurse should use clear, simple explanations.   (PED)

▶ Oral antidiabetic drugs stimulate the islets of Langerhans to produce insulin.   (M-S)

▶ Alcohol potentiates the effects of tricyclic antidepressants.   (PSY)

▶ Spontaneous rupture of the membranes increases the risk of a prolapsed umbilical cord.   (MAT)

▶ Variable decelerations are a clinical manifestation of a prolapsed umbilical cord.   (MAT)

▶ By age 3, a child should be able to stand on one foot.   (PED)

▶ *Flight of ideas* is movement from one topic to another without any discernible connection.   (PED)

▶ Most 8-month-old infants engage in imitating words.   (PED)

▶ An infant who has a congenital heart defect is at increased risk for heart failure.   (PED)

▶ Infants who have congenital heart defects are given small, frequent feedings. The typical schedule is every 3 hours instead of the usual every 4 hours.

(PED)

▶ The proper implementation for a wound evisceration is to assist the client into a supine position and cover the protruding intestine with moist, sterile saline packs. These packs are changed frequently to keep the tissue moist.   (M-S)

▶ When administering medication or other treatment to a child, the nurse should allow the child to make choices when appropriate. Making choices gives the child a sense of control over the situation and a sense of autonomy.   (PED)

▶ Milk is high in sodium and low in iron.   (FND)

▶ Conduct disorder is manifested by extreme behavior such as hurting people and animals.   (PSY)

▶ An infant who's in the learning stage of breast-feeding shouldn't be given a pacifier.   (PED)

▶ In a client with sickle cell anemia, any type of fluid loss can trigger a crisis.

(M-S)

▶ After using an inhaled corticosteroid, the client should rinse his mouth to wash away steroid residue and reduce the risk of fungal infection.   (M-S)

▶ During the tension-building phase of an abusive relationship, the abused person feels helpless.   (PSY)

▶ To build trust, an infant needs consistent care, love, and human touch. (PED)

▶ When a child is in Dunlop's traction, his body should be in alignment, especially the shoulders, hips, and legs.   (PED)

▶ In an infant, signs of impending airway obstruction include an increase in pulse and respiratory rate; substernal, suprasternal, and intercostal retractions; nasal flaring; and restlessness.   (PED)

▶ A client who has low levels of triiodothyronine and thyroxine is likely to complain of fatigue, cold intolerance, lethargy, and decreased libido.   (M-S)

▶ Treatment of a client who's in sickle cell crisis includes bed rest, hydration, restoring the electrolyte balance, and administering analgesics for pain.

(M-S)

▶ When a client expresses concern about a specific health-related issue, the nurse should assess the client's knowledge before addressing the concern.   (FND)

▶ The most effective way to reduce a fever is to administer an antipyretic, which lowers the temperature set point.   (M-S)

▶ To treat hydrocephalus, a ventriculoperitoneal shunt is placed to drain cerebrospinal fluid from the ventricles to an extracranial compartment, usually the peritoneum.   (PED)

▶ Holding his breath during a temper tantrum causes no harm to a child.
(PED)

▶ Communicating about the health needs of a family member is an essential component of meeting family needs and developing relationships.   (FND)

▶ *Ethnocentrism* is the belief that one's way of life is better than others'.   (FND)

▶ *Matiasma* is described as "bad" or "evil eye" and is said to result from envy or admiration of others.   (FND)

▶ When communicating with a non-English-speaking client through an interpreter, the nurse should speak to both the client and the interpreter, while looking at the client.   (FND)

▶ In accordance with the "hot-cold" system used by some Mexican Americans, Puerto Ricans, and other Hispanic and Latino groups, most foods, beverages, herbs, and medications are described as "cold."   (FND)

▶ *Prejudice* is a hostile attitude toward individuals of a particular group. (FND)

▶ *Discrimination* is preferential treatment of individuals of a particular group. It's usually discussed in a negative sense.   (FND)

▶ In the emergency management of a client with alcohol intoxication, his blood alcohol level is measured to determine how much medication he needs.
(PSY)

▶ If a client has respiratory alkalosis and is hyperventilating, rebreathing into a paper bag increases his partial pressure of arterial carbon dioxide.   (M-S)

▶ Adverse effects of the antidepressant fluoxetine (Prozac) include diarrhea, decreased libido, weight loss, and dry mouth.   (PSY)

▶ Chorea is a major clinical manifestation of central nervous system involvement of rheumatic fever.   (M-S)

▶ Chorea is characterized by constant jerky, uncontrolled movements of the body; mild fidgeting and twisting of the entire body; facial grimacing; and loss of bowel and bladder control.   (M-S)

▶ Before electroconvulsive therapy is performed, the skeletal muscle relaxant succinylcholine (Anectine) is given by I.V. administration.   (PSY)

▶ Severe diarrhea results in electrolyte deficiencies and metabolic acidosis.
(M-S)

▶ The most common signs and symptoms of pulmonary embolism are chest pain, dyspnea, and tachypnea.   (M-S)

▶ Children who have acute glomerulonephritis with symptoms of edema, oliguria, azotemia, and hypertension usually must restrict their dietary intake of sodium, protein, fluids, and potassium.   (PED)

▶ Increased gastric motility interferes with the absorption of oral medication. (FND)

▶ A client in labor should be turned onto her left side to relieve supine hypotension manifested by nausea, vomiting, and paleness. (MAT)

▶ To reduce the risk of hypercalcemia in a client with metastatic bone cancer, the nurse should limit his oral intake of calcium and help him ambulate. (M-S)

▶ If an infant is receiving oxygen through a nasal cannula, the nurse should monitor him for mouth breathing. (PED)

▶ Negativism is a sign of the normal growth of autonomy in a toddler. Parents should react with patience and humor and avoid head-on confrontations. (PED)

▶ The teacher, or coach, relationship is an ideal model for a positive mentoring experience. (FND)

▶ Pain associated with a myocardial infarction usually is described as pressure or a "heavy" or "squeezing" sensation in the midsternal area of the chest. The client may describe the pain as feeling as though "someone is standing on my chest" or "an elephant is standing on my chest." (M-S)

▶ When a psychotic client is admitted to an inpatient facility, the primary concern is providing safety, followed by establishing trust. (PSY)

▶ The American Academy of Pediatrics recommends introducing one food at a time to an infant and maintaining the "one-food diet" for 1 week. (PED)

▶ The first food introduced to an infant is cereal, usually rice. (PED)

▶ Calcium and phosphorus levels are elevated until hyperparathyroidism is stabilized. (M-S)

▶ Clinical evidence of coarctation of the aorta includes a bounding pulse in the arms. (FND)

▶ Resistive and challenging behaviors commonly are exhibited in the orientation phase of the therapeutic relationship. (FND)

▶ Bronchopulmonary dysplasia is an iatrogenic disease that's caused by intubation and ventilation. (PED)

▶ An infant should receive supplemental iron after age 4 months. (PED)

▶ Abdominal assessment is performed in the following order: inspection, auscultation, palpation, and percussion. (FND)

▶ An effective way to decrease the risk of suicide is to make a suicide contract with the client for a specified period. (PSY)

▶ The pain associated with carpal tunnel syndrome is caused by entrapment of the median nerve at the wrist. **(M-S)**

▶ A depressed client should be offered sufficient portions of favorite foods but shouldn't be overwhelmed by being given too much food. **(PSY)**

▶ Pancreatic enzyme replacement enhances the absorption of protein. **(M-S)**

▶ Laminectomy with spinal fusion is performed to relieve pressure on the nerves and stabilize the spine. **(M-S)**

▶ Transection injury of the spinal cord causes paralysis below the level of the lesion. **(M-S)**

▶ Toilet training can begin at 18 months. **(PED)**

▶ To allow room for other nutritious food, toddlers shouldn't consume more than 24 oz (709 ml) of milk daily. **(PED)**

▶ A child age 7 or older can use patient-controlled analgesia. **(PED)**

▶ If a spermatozoon carrying a Y chromosome fertilizes the ovum, a male zygote is formed. **(MAT)**

▶ If the ovum is fertilized by a spermatozoon carrying an X chromosome, a female zygote is formed. **(MAT)**

▶ Implantation occurs when the blastocyte implants itself in the endometrium. It usually occurs 7 to 9 days after fertilization. **(MAT)**

▶ Heart development in the embryo begins at 2 to 4 weeks and is complete by the end of the embryonic stage. **(MAT)**

▶ To determine bone age, X-rays of the tarsals and carpals are obtained to determine the degree of ossification. This technique is used primarily when the child is shorter or taller than expected, given the chronological age. **(PED)**

▶ To determine the adjusted, or correct, age of a neonate who was born prematurely, the nurse should take the chronological age and subtract the number of weeks that the infant was born prematurely. **(PED)**

▶ For a neonate, the nurse should use a blood pressure cuff that's no less than one-half and no more than two-thirds the length of the extremity that's used. **(PED)**

▶ Between the ages of 10 and 12 months, an infant should be weaned from the bottle. **(PED)**

▶ When administering oral medication to an infant, the nurse should instill the medication along the side of his tongue to prevent gagging and expulsion of the medication. **(PED)**

▶ When giving medication by Z-track injection, the nurse shouldn't use the same needle that was used to draw the medication. **(FND)**

▶ Sites for intradermal injection include the inner arm, the upper chest, and the back, under the scapula.   (FND)

▶ For pulseless ventricular tachycardia, the client should receive defibrillation immediately, beginning with 200 joules, 300 joules, and then 360 joules in rapid succession.   (M-S)

▶ Pleural friction rub is heard in pleurisy, pneumonia, and plural infarction.
                                                                                 (M-S)

▶ Wheezes are heard in emphysema, foreign-body obstruction, and asthma.
                                                                                 (M-S)

▶ Aripiprazole (Abilify) and escitalopram (Lexapro) are antipsychotic drugs used to treat schizophrenia; adverse effects include extrapyramidal reactions.
                                                                                 (PSY)

▶ Rhonchi are heard in pneumonia, emphysema, bronchitis, and bronchiectasis.
                                                                                 (M-S)

▶ Crackles are heard in pulmonary edema, pneumonia, and pulmonary fibrosis.
                                                                                 (M-S)

▶ Signs and symptoms of epiglottiditis are constant drooling, agitation (restlessness), a tripod position, and absence of spontaneous cough.   (PED)

▶ If a child has suspected epiglottiditis, the nurse shouldn't take his temperature orally or examine his throat.   (PED)

▶ Signs and symptoms of croup are hoarseness, barking (or brassy) cough, respiratory distress, and stridor.   (PED)

▶ In a client who has heart failure, the electrocardiogram shows ventricular hypertrophy.   (M-S)

▶ A crying infant must be calmed before the nurse takes his vital signs.   (PED)

▶ A 12-lead electrocardiogram should be obtained during a myocardial infarction or an anginal attack.   (M-S)

▶ The symptoms of angina can be relieved by rest or nitroglycerin. A myocardial infarction can't be relieved with rest and pain and may last 30 minutes or longer.   (M-S)

▶ Calcium channel blockers include verapamil (Calan), diltiazem (Cardizem), nifedipine (Procardia), and nicardipine (Cardene).   (M-S)

▶ Antiarrhythmic drugs include quinidine, lidocaine, and procainamide (Pronestyl).   (M-S)

▶ Angiotensin-converting enzyme inhibitors include captopril (Capoten) and enalapril (Vasotec).   (M-S)

▶ After a myocardial infarction, a client should avoid strenuous activities and stressful situations, such as exertion, extremes in temperature, and emotional stress. **(M-S)**

▶ Antihypertensive drugs include hydralazine (Apresoline) and methyldopa. **(M-S)**

▶ When evaluating whether an answer on the NCLEX is correct, consider whether the action the answer describes promotes autonomy (independence), safety, self-esteem, and a sense of belonging. **(FND)**

▶ A teenage mother may sign an informed consent for her child; it doesn't require the signature of the mother's adult parent. **(PED)**

▶ According to Piaget, between ages 2 and 7 a child is in the egocentric stage and isn't particularly concerned about rules. **(PED)**

▶ When evaluating whether an answer to a question on the NCLEX is correct, consider the cue (the stimulus for a thought) and the inference (the thought) to determine whether the inference is correct. When in doubt, select an answer that indicates the need for additional information to eliminate ambiguity. For example, a client reports that he has chest pain (the stimulus for the thought) and the nurse infers that it's cardiac pain (the thought). In this case, the nurse hasn't confirmed that the client's pain is cardiac. It would be more appropriate to make further assessments before labeling the pain as cardiac. **(FND)**

▶ *Veracity*, or truth, is an essential component of the therapeutic relationship between the health care provider and the client. **(FND)**

▶ *Beneficence* not only is the duty to do no harm but also the duty to do good. In a care setting, there's an obligation to do no harm and an equal obligation to help the client. **(FND)**

▶ *Nonmaleficence* is the duty to do no harm. **(FND)**

▶ When answering a question on the NCLEX, the basic guideline is "assess before action." Evaluate each answer carefully. Usually, several reflect the implementation phase of nursing and one or two reflect the assessment phase. In this case, an assessment response is the best choice unless there's a clear need to implement a specific course of action. **(FND)**

▶ A client with methicillin-resistant *Staphylococcus aureus* (MRSA) should be on contact isolation **(M-S)**

▶ For offspring to display the traits of a recessive gene, both parents must have the gene. **(M-S)**

▶ A third-party payer is an insurance company. **(FND)**

▶ Frye's **ABCDE** cascade provides a framework for prioritizing care by identifying the most important treatment concerns.

  A (airway)
  B (breathing)
  C (circulation)
  D (disease processes)
  E (everything else)

- **A:** The airway category includes everything that affects a patent airway, including a foreign object, fluid from an upper respiratory infection, and edema as a result of trauma or an allergic reaction.

- **B:** The breathing category includes everything that affects the breathing pattern, including hyperventilation or hypoventilation as well as abnormal breathing patterns, such as Biot's or Cheyne-Stokes respiration.

- **C:** The circulation category includes everything that affects the circulation, including fluid and electrolyte disturbances and disease processes that affect cardiac output.

- **D:** The disease processes category is assessed if the client has no problem with the airway, breathing, or circulation. The nurse should evaluate the disease processes, giving priority to the disease process that poses the greatest immediate risk. For example, in a client who has both terminal cancer and hypoglycemia, hypoglycemia is the more immediate concern.

- **E:** The everything else category includes such issues as writing an incident report and completing the client chart. When evaluating needs, this category is never the highest priority. **(FND)**

▶ *Modeling* is a form of behavior in which children imitate the behavior of a significant other such as a parent. **(FND)**

▶ *Rule utilitarianism* is known as the "greatest good for the greatest number of people" theory. **(FND)**

▶ *Egalitarian theory* emphasizes that an affluent society must provide equal access to goods and services to all, including the less fortunate. **(FND)**

▶ *Active euthanasia* is actively assisting a client to die. **(FND)**

▶ *Brain death* is irreversible cessation of all brain function. **(FND)**

▶ *Passive euthanasia* is stopping life-sustaining therapy. **(FND)**

▶ Utilization review is performed to determine whether the care provided to a client was appropriate and cost-effective. **(FND)**

▶ A *value cohort* is a group of individuals who experienced an out-of-the-ordinary event that shaped their values. **(FND)**

▶ *Voluntary euthanasia* is actively assisting the client to die at the request of the client. **(FND)**

▶ If one parent has a dominant gene, each offspring has a 50-50 chance of inheriting the gene. **(M-S)**

▶ Good sources of potassium include bananas, citrus fruits, and potatoes. **(FND)**

▶ Good sources of magnesium include fish, nuts, and grains. **(FND)**

▶ Bronchodilators dilate the bronchioles and relax the smooth muscles of the bronchioles. **(M-S)**

▶ The primary function of aldosterone is reabsorption of sodium. **(M-S)**

▶ The goal of positive end-expiratory pressure is to achieve adequate arterial oxygenation without using a toxic level of inspired oxygen or compromising cardiac output. **(M-S)**

▶ In the neonate, prolonged use of oxygen may cause retrolental fibroplasia and lead to blindness. Arterial oxygen saturation is usually maintained at less than 94%. **(PED)**

▶ Beef, oysters, shrimp, scallops, spinach, beets, and greens are good sources of iron. **(FND)**

▶ Furosemide (Lasix) is a loop diuretic. Its onset of action is 30 to 60 minutes, its peak is achieved at 1 to 2 hours, and its duration is 6 to 8 hours for the intramuscular or oral route. **(M-S)**

▶ Manual removal of fecal impaction is contraindicated in pregnancy, myocardial infarction, GI bleeding, bleeding disorders, and hemorrhoids. **(M-S)**

▶ The best method to prevent postoperative atelectasis is ambulation. Other measures include incentive spirometry and turning, coughing, and deep breathing. **(M-S)**

▶ *Intrathecal injection* is administering a drug through the spine. **(FND)**

▶ The blood urea nitrogen test and the creatinine clearance test measure how effectively the kidneys are excreting the respective substances. **(M-S)**

▶ The first sign of respiratory distress or compromise is restlessness. **(M-S)**

▶ When a question or statement by a client is emotionally charged, the nurse should respond to the emotion behind the statement or question rather than to what's said. **(FND)**

▶ The antidote for magnesium sulfate is calcium gluconate 10%. **(M-S)**

▶ A client with scarlet fever should be on respiratory isolation. The door to the client's room should be closed at all times. **(M-S)**

▶ Methergine stimulates uterine contractions. **(MAT)**

▶ Allergic reactions to blood transfusion are flushing, urticaria, wheezing, rash, chills, itching, rapid pulse, and hypotension. If any of these occurs, the nurse should stop the transfusion immediately, start the normal saline, check the client's vital signs, and notify the physician.   **(M-S)**

▶ Discharge instructions given to the parents of a child who has asthma should include instructing the child to use a peak flow meter to monitor peak expiratory flow.   **(PED)**

▶ When assessing a child who has Wilms' tumor, the nurse should avoid palpating the abdomen. A sign saying "Don't palpate abdomen" should be placed above the client's bed.   **(PED)**

▶ A client who's taking digoxin and furosemide (Lasix) should be instructed to call the physician if he experiences muscle weakness.   **(M-S)**

▶ A client who has basal cell carcinoma should be instructed to avoid sun exposure during the hottest time of the day (between 10 a.m. and 3 p.m.).   **(M-S)**

▶ Diaphoresis is a clinical manifestation of acute pain.   **(M-S)**

▶ The steps of the trajectory nursing model are:

    Step 1: Identifying the trajectory phase
    Step 2: Identifying problems and establishing goals
    Step 3: Establishing a plan to meet the goals
    Step 4: Identifying the factors that facilitate or hinder the attainment of
        goals
    Step 5: Implementing interventions
    Step 6: Evaluating the effectiveness of the interventions.   **(FND)**

▶ A Hindu client is likely to follow a vegetarian diet.   **(FND)**

▶ *Gardnerella* vaginitis is an inflammation of the vagina.   **(M-S)**

▶ Pilocarpine is a cholinergic alkaloid used as an ophthalmic miotic.   **(M-S)**

▶ If a client has a blood lead level of greater than 45 mg/dl, the physician may order chelation therapy.   **(PED)**

▶ Administering folic acid during the early stages of gestation may prevent neural tube defects.   **(MAT)**

▶ When administering metronidazole (Flagyl) to a client, the nurse should warn the client that this medicine can't be taken with alcohol because it will cause severe nausea, vomiting, and diarrhea.   **(M-S)**

▶ With advanced maternal age, a woman is more prone to conceive a baby with Down syndrome.   **(MAT)**

▶ With early maternal age, cephalopelvic disproportion commonly occurs.   **(MAT)**

▶ The client feels a tingling sensation during the administration of transcutaneous electrical nerve stimulation.   (M-S)

▶ In the early postpartum period, the fundus should be midline at the umbilicus.   (MAT)

▶ After peripheral iridectomy, postoperative care includes administering medications (steroids and cycloplegics), as prescribed, to decrease inflammation and dilate the pupils.   (M-S)

▶ One difference between acute pain and chronic pain is the pain's duration.   (FND)

▶ *Referred pain* is pain that's felt at a site other than its origin.   (FND)

▶ Initiate an incident report if clients are found engaging in sex.   (M-S)

▶ The youngest age at which it's appropriate to use the face scale to indicate the severity of pain is age 3 years.   (PED)

▶ Alleviating pain by performing a back massage is consistent with the gate-control theory.   (FND)

▶ Symptoms of retinopathy include no vision on spotty areas, seeing debris floating in the visual field, blurred vision, and diminished visual acuity.   (M-S)

▶ *Weber's test* is a bone conduction test.   (FND)

▶ *Romberg's test* is a test for balance or gait.   (FND)

▶ One treatment for trichomoniasis is metronidazole (Flagyl).   (M-S)

▶ Pain seems more intense at night because the client isn't distracted by daily activities.   (FND)

▶ A rubella vaccine shouldn't be given to a pregnant woman. It can be administered after delivery, but the client should avoid pregnancy for 3 months.   (MAT)

▶ A 16-year-old girl who's pregnant is at risk for having a low-birth-weight infant.   (MAT)

▶ A common symptom after cataract surgery is blurred vision.   (M-S)

▶ A client who has acute open-angle glaucoma may see halos around lights.   (M-S)

▶ Older clients commonly don't report pain because they fear treatment, lifestyle changes, or dependency. They also may attribute pain to aging.   (FND)

▶ To prevent otitis externa, the client should keep his ears dry when bathing.   (M-S)

▶ A long-term effect of large doses of furosemide (Lasix) administration is hearing loss.   (M-S)

▶ Before amniocentesis is performed, the mother's Rh status must be determined. **(MAT)**

▶ A complication of spinal block in a pregnant client is maternal hypotension. **(MAT)**

▶ The treatment for toxic shock syndrome is fluid and antibiotic therapy. **(M-S)**

▶ Beta-adrenergic blockers are used to treat glaucoma because they facilitate the outflow of aqueous humor. **(M-S)**

▶ No pork or pork product is allowed in a Muslim diet. **(FND)**

▶ The two goals of *Healthy People 2010* are:

1. Help individuals of all ages to increase life expectancy and improve their quality of life. **(FND)**

2. Eliminate health disparities among different segments of the population. **(FND)**

▶ A community nurse serves as a client's advocate if she tells a malnourished client to go to a meal program at a local park. **(FND)**

▶ After delivery, if the fundus is boggy and located on the right side, the client should empty her bladder. **(MAT)**

▶ A man who loses one testicle should still be able to father a child. **(M-S)**

▶ If a client isn't following his treatment plan, the nurse should first ask why. **(FND)**

▶ Falls are the leading cause of injury in elderly clients. **(FND)**

▶ Native Americans are particularly susceptible to diabetes mellitus. **(M-S)**

▶ Blacks are particularly susceptible to hypertension. **(M-S)**

▶ Cystic fibrosis is more prevalent in the white population than in the black or Hispanic population. **(M-S)**

▶ Women who are at the greatest risk for cervical cancer are those whose mothers had cervical cancer, followed by those whose sisters had cervical cancer. **(M-S)**

▶ Middle-ear hearing loss usually results from otosclerosis. **(M-S)**

▶ After testicular surgery, the client should use an ice pack for comfort. **(M-S)**

▶ *Primary prevention* is true prevention. Examples include immunizations, weight control, and smoking cessation. **(FND)**

▶ *Secondary prevention* is early detection. Examples include testing for tuberculosis, breast self-examination, testicular self-examination, and chest X-ray. **(FND)**

▶ *Tertiary prevention* is treatment to prevent long-term complications. One example is developing better treatments for cystic fibrosis. **(FND)**

▶ A client who will be providing a specimen for a sperm count should avoid ejaculation for 48 to 72 hours before the specimen is collected. **(MAT)**

▶ A client indicates that he's coming to terms with having a chronic disease when he says, "I'm never going to get any better." **(FND)**

▶ A client who has open-angle glaucoma has tunnel vision. The nurse must be careful to place items directly in front of him so that he can see them. **(M-S)**

▶ On noticing religious artifacts and literature on a client's night stand, a culturally aware nurse would ask the client what the items mean. **(FND)**

▶ A Mexican client may request the intervention of a *curandero*, or faith healer, who involves the family in his care to aid in healing. **(FND)**

▶ The hormone human chorionic gonadotropin is the marker for pregnancy. **(MAT)**

▶ Painless vaginal bleeding during the last trimester of pregnancy may indicate placenta previa. **(MAT)**

▶ Coughing with purulent sputum and fever are clinical signs of bacterial pneumonia. **(M-S)**

▶ During the transition phase of labor, the woman usually is irritable and restless. **(MAT)**

▶ Signs and symptoms of flail chest include paradoxical movements of the involved chest wall, dyspnea, pain, and cyanosis. **(M-S)**

▶ Right-sided cardiac function is assessed by evaluating central venous pressure. **(M-S)**

▶ A client who has a pacemaker should report immediately an increase or decrease in the pulse rate of more than 4 to 5 beats/minute. **(M-S)**

▶ Dizziness, fainting, palpitation, hiccups, and chest pain indicate pacemaker failure, and the physician should be notified if these occur. **(M-S)**

▶ Leukemia causes easy fatigability, generalized malaise, pallor, and shortness of breath on activity. **(M-S)**

▶ After cardiac catheterization, the puncture, or cutdown, site should be monitored for hematoma formation. **(M-S)**

▶ Estriol levels are measured to assess fetal well-being most commonly in pregnancies complicated by diabetes. **(MAT)**

▶ A client with pancytopenia should be on reverse isolation. **(M-S)**

▶ If the nurse notices water in a ventilator tube, she should remove the water from the tube and reconnect it. **(M-S)**

▶ Tamoxifen is an antineoplastic drug that's used to treat breast cancer.　(M-S)

▶ The adverse effects of vincristine (Oncovin) include alopecia, nausea, and vomiting.　(M-S)

▶ To avoid puncturing the placenta, a vaginal examination shouldn't be performed on a pregnant client who's bleeding.　(MAT)

▶ A client who has postpartum hemorrhage caused by uterine atony should be given oxytocin as prescribed.　(MAT)

▶ Emphysema is characterized by destruction of the alveoli, enlargement of the distal air spaces, and breakdown of the alveolar walls.　(M-S)

▶ To keep secretions thin, the client who has emphysema should increase his fluid intake.　(M-S)

▶ The signs and symptoms of asthma are wheezing, dyspnea, hypoxemia, diaphoresis, and increased heart and respiratory rate.　(M-S)

▶ *Extrinsic asthma* is an antigen–antibody reaction to such allergens as pollen, animal dander, feathers, foods, house dust, or mites.　(M-S)

▶ Laceration of the vagina, cervix, or perineum produces bright red bleeding that typically comes in spurts. The bleeding is continuous, even when the fundus is firm.　(MAT)

▶ To stimulate the rooting reflex and promote feeding, the nurse should stroke the infant's cheek.　(PED)

▶ After endoscopy is performed, the nurse should assess the client for hemoptysis.　(M-S)

▶ Increased urine output is an indication that a hypertensive crisis has resolved.　(M-S)

▶ After radical mastectomy, the client should be positioned with the affected arm placed on pillows. The hand should be elevated and aligned with the arm.　(M-S)

▶ After pneumonectomy, the client should perform arm exercises to prevent frozen shoulder.　(M-S)

▶ Right-sided heart failure causes edema, distended neck veins, nocturia, and weakness.　(M-S)

▶ Left-sided heart failure causes crackles, coughing, tachycardia, and fatigability.　(M-S)

▶ Cardiac glycosides increase contractility and cardiac output.　(M-S)

▶ Adverse effects of cardiac glycosides include cardiac disturbance, headache, hypotension, GI symptoms, blurred vision, and yellow-green halos around lights.　(M-S)

▶ A client who's receiving anticoagulant therapy should take acetaminophen (Tylenol) instead of aspirin for pain. (M-S)

▶ Adequate humidification is important after laryngectomy. At home, the client can use pans of water or a cool mist vaporizer, especially in the bedroom. (M-S)

▶ Late symptoms of renal cancer include hematuria, flank pain, and a palpable mass in the flank. (M-S)

▶ When heparin is given subcutaneously, it's usually given in the lower abdominal fat pad. (M-S)

▶ In a client who has sickle cell anemia, warm packs should be placed over the extremities to relieve pain. Cold packs may stimulate vasoconstriction and cause further ischemia. The extremities also should be placed on pillows for comfort. (M-S)

▶ Sickle cell crisis causes sepsis (fever greater than 102° F [38.9° C], meningeal irritation, tachypnea, tachycardia, and hypotension) and vaso-occlusive crisis (severe pain) with hypoxemia (partial pressure of arterial oxygen of less than 70 mm Hg). (M-S)

▶ In an infant, the normal hemoglobin value is 12 g/dl. (M-S)

▶ Adverse effects of digoxin include headache, weakness, vision disturbances, anorexia, and GI upset. (M-S)

▶ To perform a tuberculosis test, a 26G needle is used with a 1-ml syringe. (M-S)

▶ The nitrogen balance estimates the difference between the intake and utilization of protein. (FND)

▶ Respiratory failure occurs when mucus blocks the alveoli or the airways of the lungs. (M-S)

▶ The client should be instructed not to cough during thoracentesis. (M-S)

▶ Hot compresses can reduce breast tenderness after breast-feeding. (MAT)

▶ A client who has thrombophlebitis should be placed in the Trendelenburg position. (M-S)

▶ Symptoms of Pneumocystis jiroveci (carinii) pneumonia—common in clients with AIDS—include dyspnea and nonproductive cough. (M-S)

▶ To counteract vitamin B_1 deficiency, a client who has pernicious anemia should eat meat and animal products. (M-S)

▶ A client who's on a ventilator and becomes restless should undergo suctioning. (M-S)

▶ A premature neonate has a decrease in surfactant that leads to decreased oxygen consumption. (PED)

▶ Autologous bone marrow transplantation doesn't cause graft-versus-host disease. (M-S)

▶ A client who has mild thrombophlebitis is likely to have mild cramping on exertion. (M-S)

▶ If the first attempt to perform colostomy irrigation is unsuccessful, the procedure is repeated with normal saline. (M-S)

▶ The fundus of a postpartum client is massaged to stimulate contraction of the uterus and prevent hemorrhage. (MAT)

▶ Breast enlargement in men or boys, or *gynecomastia*, is an adverse effect of estrogen therapy. (M-S)

▶ In a client with leukemia, a low platelet count may lead to hemorrhage. (M-S)

▶ After radical neck dissection, the immediate concern is respiratory distress as a result of tracheal edema. (M-S)

▶ Naloxone (Narcan) is given to a neonate who's experiencing the effects of maternal opioid administration during labor and delivery. (PED)

▶ In a neonate who's large for gestational age, the serum glucose level should be measured. (PED)

▶ A mother who has a positive human immunodeficiency virus test result shouldn't breast-feed her infant. (MAT)

▶ After radical mastectomy, the client's arm should be positioned over the table and supported with a pillow to prevent lymphedema. (M-S)

▶ Hypoventilation causes respiratory acidosis. (M-S)

▶ The high Fowler position promotes better breathing for a client who has orthopnea. (M-S)

▶ To obtain a urine specimen in an infant, the nurse uses a specimen bag (Hollister U bag). (PED)

▶ A transient ischemic attack affects sensory and motor function and may cause diplopia, dysphagia, aphasia, and ataxia. (M-S)

▶ After mastectomy, the client should squeeze a ball with the hand on the affected side. (M-S)

▶ Cholestyramine (Questran), which is used to reduce the serum cholesterol level, may cause constipation. (M-S)

▶ Dinoprostone (Cervidil) is used to ripen the cervix. (MAT)

▶ Glucocorticoid, or steroid, therapy may mask the signs of infection. (M-S)

▶ After the death of a child, the parents should be allowed to stay with the child for as long as they wish. **(PED)**

▶ Breast-feeding of a premature neonate born at 32 weeks' gestation can be accomplished if the mother expresses milk and feeds the infant by gavage. **(PED)**

▶ Melanoma is most commonly seen in light-skinned people who work or spend time outdoors. **(M-S)**

▶ A client who has a pacemaker should take his pulse at the same time every day. **(M-S)**

▶ A client who has stomatitis should rinse his mouth with mouthwash frequently. **(M-S)**

▶ An adverse effect of theophylline administration is tachycardia. **(M-S)**

▶ The treatment for laryngotracheobronchitis includes postural drainage before meals. **(M-S)**

▶ After radical neck dissection, a high priority is providing a means of communication. **(M-S)**

▶ A high-fat diet that includes red meat is a contributing factor for colorectal cancer. **(M-S)**

▶ After a modified radical mastectomy, the client should be placed in the semi-Fowler position, with the arm placed on a pillow. **(M-S)**

▶ A young child is sedated before cardiac catheterization is performed. **(PED)**

▶ Knifelike, stabbing pain in the chest suggests pulmonary embolism. **(M-S)**

▶ Esophageal cancer is associated with excessive alcohol consumption. **(M-S)**

▶ If a pregnant client's rubella titer is less than 1:8, she should be immunized after delivery. **(MAT)**

▶ The administration of oxytocin (Pitocin) is stopped if the contractions are 90 seconds or longer. **(MAT)**

▶ For an extramural delivery (one that takes place outside of a normal delivery center), the priorities for care of the neonate include maintaining a patent airway, supporting efforts to breathe, monitoring vital signs, and maintaining adequate body temperature. **(MAT)**

▶ When an infant receives phototherapy with a fiber-optic light, it isn't necessary to cover the eyes or genitals. **(PED)**

▶ A client who has pancytopenia and is undergoing chemotherapy may develop hemorrhage and infection. **(M-S)**

▶ A grade I tumor is encapsulated and grows by expansion. **(M-S)**

▶ Subinvolution may occur if the bladder is distended after delivery.　(MAT)

▶ The nurse must place identification bands on both the mother and the neonate before they leave the delivery room.　(MAT)

▶ Cancer of the pancreas causes anorexia, weight loss, and jaundice.　(M-S)

▶ To reduce the risk of dumping syndrome after gastric surgery, the client should lie down for 30 to 45 minutes after meals.　(M-S)

▶ Most water absorption occurs in the large intestine.　(FND)

▶ Most nutrients are absorbed in the small intestine.　(FND)

▶ Prolonged gastric suctioning can cause metabolic alkalosis.　(M-S)

▶ To measure the amount of residual urine, the nurse performs straight catheterization after the client voids.　(M-S)

▶ Dexamethasone (Decadron) is a steroidal anti-inflammatory agent that's used to treat brain tumors.　(M-S)

▶ Long-term reduction in the delivery of oxygen to the kidneys causes an increase in erythropoiesis.　(M-S)

▶ When assessing a client's eating habits, the nurse should ask, "What have you eaten in the last 24 hours?"　(FND)

▶ A vegan diet includes an abundant supply of fiber.　(FND)

▶ To facilitate emptying of the stomach after feeding, the infant is positioned on his right side.　(PED)

▶ A client who subsists on canned foods and canned fish is at risk for sodium imbalance, or hypernatremia.　(M-S)

▶ Clinical signs and symptoms of hypoxia include confusion, diaphoresis, changes in blood pressure, tachycardia, and tachypnea.　(M-S)

▶ Red meat can cause a false-positive result on a fecal occult blood test.　(M-S)

▶ Carbon monoxide replaces hemoglobin in the red blood cells, decreasing the amount of oxygen in the tissue.　(M-S)

▶ A client who has alkaline urine can be predisposed to a urinary tract infection.　(M-S)

▶ A hypotonic enema softens the feces, distends the colon, and stimulates peristalsis.　(FND)

▶ Bladder retraining is effective if it lengthens the intervals between urination.　(M-S)

▶ *Cheilosis,* or cracks in the corner of the mouth, is caused by riboflavin deficiency.　(M-S)

▶ First-morning urine provides the best specimen to measure glucose, ketone, pH, and specific gravity values.   (FND)

▶ The concentration of oxygen in inspired air is reduced at high altitudes. As a result, dyspnea may occur on exertion.   (M-S)

▶ A client who's receiving enteric feeding should be assessed for abdominal distention.   (M-S)

▶ Thiamine deficiency causes neuropathy.   (M-S)

▶ A client who has abdominal distention as a result of flatus may be treated with a carminative enema (Harris flush).   (M-S)

▶ Pernicious anemia is caused by a deficiency of vitamin B_{12}, or cobalamin.
                                                                                (M-S)

▶ After a barium enema, the client is given a laxative.   (M-S)

▶ The appropriate I.V. fluid to correct a hypovolemic, or fluid volume, deficit is normal saline solution.   (M-S)

▶ Serum albumin deficiency is common in clients with burn injuries.   (M-S)

▶ Before giving a gastrostomy feeding, the nurse should inspect the stoma.
                                                                                (M-S)

▶ After a laminectomy, the client should be logrolled to reposition.   (M-S)

▶ Hyponatremia may occur in a client who has a high fever and drinks only water.   (M-S)

▶ Folic acid deficiency causes muscle weakness as a result of hypoxemia. (M-S)

▶ Disorientation, tachycardia, and hypotension are clinical signs of dehydration.
                                                                                (M-S)

▶ To induce sleep, the first step is to minimize environmental stimuli.   (FND)

▶ Before moving a client, the nurse should assess the client's physical abilities and ability to understand instructions as well as the amount of strength required to move the client.   (FND)

▶ If a child is having difficulty falling asleep, the nurse should maintain the child's bedtime ritual, such as reading a story or holding a favorite blanket or toy.   (PED)

▶ Glucocorticoids can cause an electrolyte imbalance.   (M-S)

▶ A decrease in potassium level decreases the effectiveness of cardiac glycosides, increases possible digoxin toxicity, and can cause fatal cardiac arrhythmia.
                                                                                (M-S)

▶ Diuresis can cause decreased absorption of vitamins A, D, E, and K.   (M-S)

▶ Protein depletion causes a decrease in lymphocyte count.   (M-S)

▶ If they're old enough, children may be given popcorn to alleviate constipation. **(PED)**

▶ To lose 1 lb (0.5 kg) in 1 week, the client must decrease his intake by 3,500 calories (about 500 calories per day). To lose 2 lb (1 kg) in 1 week, the client must decrease his caloric intake by 7,000 calories (about 1,000 calories per day). **(FND)**

▶ To prevent paraphimosis after the insertion of a Foley catheter, the nurse should replace the prepuce. **(M-S)**

▶ To avoid shearing force injury, a client who's completely immobile is lifted on a sheet. **(FND)**

▶ Loop diuretics, such as furosemide (Lasix), decrease plasma levels of potassium and sodium. **(M-S)**

▶ After excretory urography, the client should drink plenty of fluids to promote the excretion of dye. **(M-S)**

▶ Potassium should be taken with food and fluids. **(M-S)**

▶ To insert a catheter from the nose through the trachea for suction, the nurse should ask the client to swallow. **(FND)**

▶ Proper measurement of a nasogastric tube is from the corner of the mouth to the ear lobe to the tip of the sternum. **(FND)**

▶ Vitamin C is needed for collagen production in wound healing. **(FND)**

▶ A client who has Addison's disease and is receiving corticosteroid therapy is at increased risk for infection. **(M-S)**

▶ To assess a client for hemorrhage after a thyroidectomy, the nurse should roll the client to the side to examine the sides and back of the neck. **(M-S)**

▶ A client who's receiving hormone therapy for hypothyroidism should take the medication at the same time each day. **(M-S)**

▶ Hyperproteinemia may contribute to the development of hepatic encephalopathy. **(M-S)**

▶ To minimize bleeding in a client who has liver dysfunction, small-gauge needles are used for injections. **(M-S)**

▶ A client who has cirrhosis of the liver and ascites should follow a low-sodium diet. **(M-S)**

▶ Before excretory urography, the nurse must ask the client whether he's allergic to iodine or shellfish. **(M-S)**

▶ A *buffalo hump* is an abnormal distribution of adipose tissue that occurs in Cushing's syndrome. **(M-S)**

▶ Levothyroxine (Synthroid) is used as replacement therapy in hypothyroidism.
(M-S)

▶ Acne vulgaris, one result of the hormonal changes of adolescence, is caused by androgenic stimulation of sebum production. (PED)

▶ Levothyroxine (Synthroid) treats, but doesn't cure, hypothyroidism and must be taken for the client's lifetime. It shouldn't be taken with food because food may interfere with its absorption. (M-S)

▶ Imipramine (Tofranil) with concomitant use of barbiturates or central nervous system (CNS) depressants will result in enhanced CNS depression.
(M-S)

▶ A client who's receiving levothyroxine (Synthroid) therapy should report tachycardia to the physician. (M-S)

▶ The signs and symptoms of hyperkalemia include muscle weakness, hypotension, shallow respiration, apathy, and anorexia. (M-S)

▶ In a client who has well-controlled diabetes, the 2-hour postprandial blood glucose level may be 139 mg/dl. (M-S)

▶ A client who has diabetes mellitus should wash his feet daily in warm water and dry them carefully, especially between the toes. (M-S)

▶ Acute pancreatitis causes constant epigastric abdominal pain that radiates to the back and flank and is more intense in the supine position. (M-S)

▶ A client who's receiving lithium (Eskalith) therapy should report diarrhea, vomiting, drowsiness, muscular weakness, or lack of coordination to the physician immediately. The therapeutic serum level for maintenance is 0.6 to 1.2 mEq/L. (PSY)

▶ Obsessive–compulsive disorder is an anxiety-based disorder. (PSY)

▶ Al-Anon is a self-help group for families of alcoholics. (PSY)

▶ Signs and symptoms of acute respiratory distress syndrome include dyspnea, cyanosis, rhonchi, restlessness, and decreased breath sounds. (M-S)

▶ After electroconvulsive therapy, the client is placed in the lateral position, with his head turned to one side. (PSY)

▶ The triple screen is performed at 15 to 20 weeks' gestation to identify such complications as Down syndrome and neural tube defects. (MAT)

▶ Giving away personal possessions is a sign of suicidal ideation. Other signs include writing a suicide note and talking about suicide. (PSY)

▶ Toddlers are more susceptible to lead poisoning than adults because of pica and because they are closer to ground dust that's being kicked up. (PED)

▶ Oral hypoglycemic agents are contraindicated during pregnancy because of possible adverse effects on the fetus and newborn. **(MAT)**

▶ Diabetic neuropathy is a long-term complication of diabetes mellitus. **(M-S)**

▶ To assess a client's judgment, the nurse should ask the client what he would do if he found a stamped, addressed envelope. An appropriate response is that he would mail the envelope. **(PSY)**

▶ After electroconvulsive therapy, the client should be monitored for postshock amnesia. **(PSY)**

▶ A mother who continues to perform cardiopulmonary resuscitation after a physician pronounces a child dead is exhibiting denial. **(PSY)**

▶ *Transvestism* is a desire to wear clothes commonly worn by members of the opposite sex. **(PSY)**

▶ Portal vein hypertension is associated with liver cirrhosis. **(M-S)**

▶ After thyroidectomy, the nurse should assess the client for laryngeal damage that's manifested by hoarseness. **(M-S)**

▶ The client with hypoparathyroidism has hypocalcemia. **(M-S)**

▶ Tardive dyskinesia produces excessive blinking, unusual movements of the tongue, and involuntary sucking and chewing. It's caused by long-term use of antipsychotic drugs. **(PSY)**

▶ Trihexyphenidyl hydrochloride (Artane) and benztropine mesylate (Cogentin) are administered to counteract extrapyramidal effects. **(PSY)**

▶ To prevent hypertensive crisis, a client who's taking a monoamine oxidase inhibitor should avoid consuming aged cheese, caffeine, beer, yeast, chocolate, liver, processed foods, and monosodium glutamate. **(PSY)**

▶ Extrapyramidal symptoms include parkinsonism, dystonia, akathisia ("ants in the pants"), and tardive dyskinesia. **(PSY)**

▶ A client who has chronic pancreatitis should consume a bland, low-fat diet. **(M-S)**

▶ A client with hepatitis A should be on enteric precautions to prevent the spread of hepatitis A. **(M-S)**

▶ The client who has liver disease is likely to have jaundice, which is caused by an increased bilirubin level. **(M-S)**

▶ An adverse effect of phenytoin (Dilantin) administration is hyperplasia of the gingiva. **(M-S)**

▶ Protein intake must be monitored in the child who has phenylketonuria. **(PED)**

▶ Hematemesis is a clinical sign of esophageal varices. **(M-S)**

▶ Fat destruction is the chemical process that causes ketones to appear in urine.
(M-S)

▶ One theory that supports the use of electroconvulsive therapy suggests that it "resets" the brain circuits to allow normal function.
(PSY)

▶ A client with sickle cell anemia should receive oxygen only briefly because long-term use interferes with bone marrow activity and aggravates the condition.
(M-S)

▶ A client who has obsessive-compulsive disorder usually recognizes the senselessness of his behavior but is powerless to stop it (ego-dystonia).
(PSY)

▶ *Atelectasis* and *dehiscence* are postoperative conditions associated with removal of the gallbladder.
(M-S)

▶ After liver biopsy, the client should be positioned on the right side, with a pillow placed underneath the liver border.
(M-S)

▶ In helping a client who has been abused, physical safety is the nurse's first priority.
(PSY)

▶ Pemoline (Cylert) is used to treat attention deficit hyperactivity disorder (ADHD).
(PSY)

▶ Before thyroidectomy, Lugol's solution is used to devascularize the gland.
(M-S)

▶ Clozapine (Clozaril) is contraindicated in pregnant women and in clients who have severe granulocytopenia or severe central nervous system depression.
(M-S)

▶ Cholecystitis causes low-grade fever, nausea, vomiting, guarding of the right upper quadrant, and biliary pain that radiates to the right scapula.
(M-S)

▶ Early symptoms of liver cirrhosis include fatigue, anorexia, edema of the ankles in the evening, epistaxis, and bleeding gums.
(M-S)

▶ Iron tablets should be stored out of the reach of children.
(M-S)

▶ Don't give iron with milk products because they interfere with iron absorption.
(M-S)

▶ The signs and symptoms of diabetes insipidus include polydipsia, polyuria, specific gravity of 1.001 to 1.005, and high serum osmolality.
(M-S)

▶ Hypnosis is used to treat psychogenic amnesia.
(PSY)

▶ Hypertension is a sign of rejection of a transplanted kidney.
(M-S)

▶ Lactulose is used to prevent and treat portal-systemic encephalopathy.
(M-S)

▶ A child's failure to grow above the third percentile by age 2 years may be related to hypopituitarism.
(PED)

▶ Extracorporeal and intracorporeal shock wave lithotripsy is the use of shock waves to perform noninvasive destruction of biliary stones. It's indicated in the treatment of symptomatic high-risk clients who have few noncalcified cholesterol stones. **(M-S)**

▶ Disulfiram (Antabuse) is administered orally as an aversion therapy to treat alcoholism. **(PSY)**

▶ Ingestion of alcohol by a client who's taking disulfiram (Antabuse) causes severe reactions, including nausea and vomiting, and may endanger the life of the client. **(PSY)**

▶ Signs and symptoms of congenital dislocation of the hip include gluteal folds, with deeper creases apparent on the affected side, and limited hip abduction on the affected side, which produces a click (Ortolani click). **(PED)**

▶ Cretinism is suspected when the mother reports that her baby sleeps all the time and doesn't cry. He may be described as a "good baby." **(PED)**

▶ Decreased consciousness is a clinical sign of an increased ammonia level. **(M-S)**

▶ Clients who have acute pancreatitis receive meperidine (Demerol) for pain. **(M-S)**

▶ Prochlorperazine (Compazine), meclizine (Antivert), and trimethobenzamide (Tigan) are used to treat the nausea and vomiting caused by cholecystitis. **(M-S)**

▶ Improved concentration is a sign that lithium is taking effect. **(PSY)**

▶ Behavior modification, including time outs, token economy, and a reward system, is a treatment for attention deficit hyperactivity disorder. **(PSY)**

▶ Magnesium is found in green, leafy vegetables and whole grains. **(FND)**

▶ Milk and milk products, poultry, grains, and fish are good sources of phosphate. **(FND)**

▶ Cryoprecipitate contains factors VIII and XIII and fibrinogen and is used to treat hemophilia. **(M-S)**

▶ A walker should be advanced, together with the weaker leg, about 6" (15 cm) at a time. **(FND)**

▶ Insomnia is the most common sleep disorder. **(M-S)**

▶ Cerebral palsy is a nonprogressive disorder. Treatment is intended to help the child maximize his potential. **(PED)**

▶ The major function of sodium in the body is to regulate the amount of fluid the body contains. **(FND)**

▶ The best way to prevent falls at night in an oriented but restless elderly client is to raise the bed's side rails. (FND)

▶ In the working phase of the nurse-client relationship, the nurse helps the client to explore his thoughts, feelings, and actions and to plan a program of action to meet the established goals. (FND)

▶ By the end of the orientation phase, the client should begin to trust the nurse. (FND)

▶ Listening is the most effective communication technique to use with a child who stutters. (PED)

▶ Falls in the elderly are likely to be caused by poor vision. (FND)

▶ The health continuum is best described as a constant state of change. (FND)

▶ Barriers to communication include language deficits, sensory deficits, cognitive impairments, structural deficits, and paralysis. (FND)

▶ A client who's receiving a hypnotic medication may experience a decrease in rapid-eye-movement sleep but an overall increase in sleep. (FND)

▶ The lateral position should be used to administer oral hygiene to an unconscious client. (FND)

▶ The three elements that are necessary for a fire are heat, oxygen, and combustible material. (FND)

▶ A sitz bath is effective when it lessens pain and stimulates circulation. (FND)

▶ Clients who have diabetes should file their toenails straight across. (M-S)

▶ Smoking is a maladaptive response to stress. (FND)

▶ Elderly clients are at risk for osteoporosis because of age-related bone demineralization. (M-S)

▶ To check for petechiae in a dark-skinned client, the nurse should assess the oral mucosa. (FND)

▶ The signs and symptoms of local infection in an extremity are tenderness, loss of use of the extremity, erythema, edema, and warmth. (M-S)

▶ Signs and symptoms of systemic infection include fever and swollen lymph nodes. (M-S)

▶ Opisthotonos (abnormal posture) is a sign of meningitis. (FND)

▶ An immobile client is predisposed to thrombus formation because of increased blood stasis. (M-S)

▶ To increase client comfort, the nurse should let the alcohol dry before giving an I.M. injection. (FND)

▶ Treatment for a stage I ulcer on the heels includes heel protectors. (FND)

▶ Treatment for stomatitis includes oral care. (M-S)

▶ Sources of vitamin C include potatoes, citrus fruits, cantaloupe, and green peppers. (FND)

▶ Seventh-Day Adventists are usually vegetarians. (FND)

▶ Lean, tender meat, fish, and poultry can be served as part of a soft diet. (FND)

▶ Urea is the chief end product of amino acid metabolism. (M-S)

▶ Morphine and other opioids relieve pain by binding to the nerve cells in the dorsal horn of the spinal cord. (M-S)

▶ Endorphins are morphinelike substances that produce a feeling of well-being. (FND)

▶ *Pain tolerance* is the maximum amount of pain an individual is willing to endure. (FND)

▶ Full agonist analgesics include morphine, codeine, meperidine (Demerol), propoxyphene (Darvon), and hydromorphone (Dilaudid). (M-S)

▶ Buprenorphine (Buprenex) is a partial agonist analgesic. (M-S)

▶ Cutaneous stimulation causes the release of endorphins that block the transmission of pain stimuli. (FND)

▶ *Trichomonas* and *Candida* infections can be acquired nonsexually. (M-S)

▶ A client with cystic fibrosis shouldn't be given cough syrup or antihistamines because his cough shouldn't be suppressed. (M-S)

Index

183